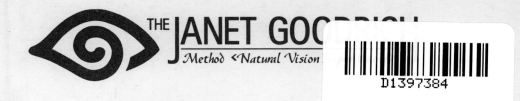

THE JANET GOODRICH
Method ‹Natural Vision

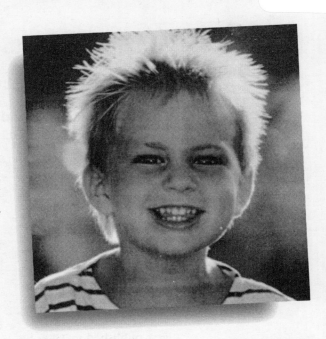

Help your child to perfect eyesight without glasses

By Janet Goodrich
MILNER

This book is for my beloved father,
Sidney Marcellus Goodrich.

First published in 1996 by

Sally Milner Publishing Pty Ltd
RMB 54 Burra Road,
Burra Creek NSW 2620
Australia

© Janet Goodrich, 1996

Design by Design One, Sydney
Printed and bound by Australian Print Group, Maryborough,
Victoria, Australia

Cataloguing-in-Publication Data

Goodrich, Janet.
Helping your child to perfect eyesight without glasses.

Bibliography.
Includes index.
ISBN 1 86351 194 6.

1. Vision. 2. Visual training. 3. Vision disorders in
children. I. Title.

618.92097

Dear Reader,

Did your heart sink when you saw the report: 'Your child's eyesight has been tested and found lacking. Please take him to an optometrist for an exam and glasses'? Do you still sigh and resign yourself to the sight of your bright-eyed toddler locked forever into a blurred world after a year or two in school? Does hearing that ever-thicker glasses are normal and necessary make you grind your teeth?

Now you, a mere parent or grandparent, armed with only love and willingness, can turn a faulty vision report into a blazing adventure and miniature miracle for yourself and your child.

By taking one step at a time through this book, you and your whole family will gain a deeper understanding of the causes of blurred vision. Walking natural pathways to restoring clarity of eyesight will allow you to drop the crutches of optical devices along your way.

Rational explanations and insights are followed by a host of practical, easy vision improvement games. Using and reusing this book will lighten your heart and get that child out of glasses!

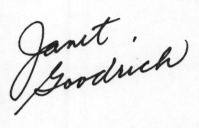

Janet Goodrich

Janet Goodrich has a doctorate in psychology. From 1975 to 1983 she directed the Vital Health Centre in Los Angeles. In 1990 she established her Instructor Training Centre for Natural Vision Improvement near Brisbane, Australia. For over 20 years she has taught her method in the USA, Australia, England, Switzerland, Germany and Asia. Since 1992 she has been creating methods and seminars for naturally improving children's eyesight.

United Syndicate and Plenum Press kindly allowed reprint of copyrighted materials. All efforts have been made to contact other original copyright holders . Any discrepancies will be altered upon notice. Thanks to the family of Helen M. Kennedy for giving her Corbett materials to Janet Goodrich.

Illustrations: Veronica Davidson. Page 119 Fiona Whipp, pages 111 and 176 Chris Dent, page 191 Louise Coutts.

Cover photo: Jean-Paul Nacivet, Author photo: Steven Lang. Page 119 S. Fredlyand

All other photos by Janet Goodrich or from her personal archives. Book Design: Design One Graphics Pty. Ltd.

Technical consultants: Optometrists Adrian Bell , Bryan Smith and Ross Fisher

Contents

👁 Help Your Child to Perfect Eyesight

Chapter Seven   Vision is alive and well in the brain

Chapter Eight   Eyes must move to see   89

Part Four   Home and School Environments

11

Natural Vision Improvement is an educational programme. The author of this book is not directly or indirectly representing this material as diagnosis or prescription for any ailment. If you suspect a medical condition please visit a licensed doctor. Use of the procedures described here is entirely at the reader's own risk. Any positive results you obtain from using this material are your responsibility and to your own credit.

Why I wrote this book

Ordinary citizens are longing to be directly active in preventing and reversing eyesight problems. Trained professionals are seeking a more human way of working with eyesight.

My suitcases were standing in the doorway, heavy with papers and books for the coming Teacher Training course in Germany. The phone rang. A woman in Newcastle described her nine-month-old grandson trying to crawl about the living-room with glasses taped to his head and one eye covered with plaster. 'It breaks my heart,' she said. 'Is there anything I can do to help him?'

Following my lecture in London at the Alternative Medicine Festival, a woman who does fusion training with children after strabismus operations grabbed my hand and moaned, 'I have ten minutes with each baby. I really want to do something more with these children'.

Upon arriving home I found a letter from Malaysia on my desk. An eight year-old boy had just received his second pair of glasses within one year. His prescription had jumped from -5 to -8 diopters. Progressive myopia was the diagnosis, stronger glasses the only response. 'Where will it end?' his mother wondered. In 1993 the government in Singapore spent thousands of dollars installing better lighting in classrooms, hoping somehow to hold back the tidal wave of myopia that sweeps 57 percent of all teenage boys in that country into glasses.

It is obvious that the automatic response of putting glasses on any child who manifests visual blur isn't helping. The possible causes of poor eyesight are ignored. Parents are left out of the picture altogether, except as cheque-writers and enforcers of the 'make her wear them all the time' rule. Most children's lifestyle, schooling, and diet are determined by mass marketing and cultural habits. Meanwhile you, as the producer and constant care-giver of the child, are written off as a dummy who should blindly obey the command:

'Take the children for earlier and more frequent eye exams. But don't attempt any home remedies because you don't know enough.'

The continuing frustration and apathy generated by the established optical industry challenged me and my myopic childhood. I had proudly sprouted glasses at age seven for myopia and astigmatism.

After 20 years behind coke-bottle-thick lenses my inner being said, 'Enough'. Having used the Natural Vision Improvement processes myself I discarded the glasses at age 27, passed all my vision tests without visual aids of any kind and began to teach others to do the same. This child who shielded herself for 20 years behind a pair of glasses is tuning into every child on this planet. She said 'Write!' - for the children who are going myopic, hyperopic and cross-eyed. She said, 'Tell parents children don't have to be put in glasses.'

Social and optical pressures

The dimming of once bright, sharp eyes is a signal to interact with your child. The artificial clarity of robot-goggles obscures the constant opportunities to lead children toward naturally clear vision.

The pressure to use an optical solution is pervasive in our culture. Every day you will be confronted in your endeavour by voices and visuals denying the power to heal eyesight with natural means. Every shopping plaza sports an eyewear boutique. School teachers have curriculum standards to maintain, tests to administer and criticisms to bear. These good people are anxious to make sure the child performs well. Glasses, everyone knows, are required for adequate performance in the classroom. Grown-ups are relieved when the child can finally see and enjoy reading. Yet the signal flares are dulled. The glasses keep getting stronger. Cause is locked away in a back closet.

Be ready to deal with the disdain and patronising righteousness of the optical experts. These folk are both well-meaning and trapped in their expensive training. Only licensed practitioners may diagnose the condition of the eye and determine the function of the visual apparatus of the human body. However what you do with the diagnosis is up to you. You will probably hear, 'There's nothing you can do to change this child's vision, except...' Interpret this as: 'There is nothing I can do to change this child's vision except...' Do not let authoritarian opinions deter you. Imagine being a mouse eavesdropping on a conference open only to licensed doctors. You'd probably hear angry voices and the clash of one 'scientific' belief system against another.

A new Attitude

Many optometrists and even ophthalmologists have changed their minds about Natural Vision Improvement, using it themselves and recommending it to their patients.

"I hold Janet Goodrich's book in my hand with delight and gratitude. It is an honour. A few years ago I would have rejected it out of hand. What I had learned in medical school was gospel. There are problems that can be healed and other that cannot. But the causes of the latter were all unknown, and I was not open to the possibility that 'concrete facts' could be seen from another angle. Through my own experience I was led into another world, a new world of health and energy. On the non-physical level powerful influences are active that orthodox medicine cannot reach. Often 'incurable' illnesses disappear.

I wish from my heart that many people will use the playful and potent ideas in this book. Parents can sow many beneficial seeds for their children's vision while walking new and enjoyable pathways together."

Editha Neumann, ophthalmologist, Germany

"We are living in times of great change. ...many people are increasingly dissatisfied with mechanical medicine and are deeply affected by the lack of time for explanation and human warmth from doctors. The great interest in alternative, gentler forms of therapy that speak to one's inner experience is growing accordingly.

The solution does not lie in 'either-or'. A valid answer comes only through a synthesis of both approaches. Janet Goodrich's book is a step in the right direction. Even established conservative eye doctors are beginning to see that the eye cannot be treated adequately when separated from mental and emotional considerations.

We ophthalmologists would do neither ourselves nor our patients a favour by rejecting the whole person approach to vision in this book. The adage holds, 'Whoever heals is right.' Too often we assume that the previous measurements made by a colleague or optometrist were totally accurate. Every day in practice I encounter unexplainable changes in vision. Other areas of the body heal without mechanical intervention; why not eyesight?

I believe that this book, based on the author's many years of experience, offers everyone food for thought and valuable ways our patients can be helped, rather than prescribing yet another pair of glasses.

Joy Patricia Wermann, ophthalmologist, Germany

"I am honoured to write about this book. In the rising chorus of voices criticizing traditional ophthalmological and optometric treatment of functional vision problems, the voice of Janet Goodrich is worth listening to and has a clear message.

Consistent with well-documented vision research, Janet Goodrich presents an elucidating educational progamme. She speaks of the dynamic interplay between the child's eyes and the environment. In Janet's Method, mechanical devices—glasses and machinery, are used as little as possible. Her emphasis is on reconnecting the child (and the child within all of us) to the resources of life-energy that are inherent in a joyful, exploring youth. These are the powerful resources that are obstructed during everyday life by the demands imposed on us all by education and society.

Our visual system is affected by every thought we think, the emotions we feel and the movements we make. Twenty percent of the optic nerve fibres connect the light impulses coming from the eye to neural centres of attention, emotion, body tone, movement and posture. Our eyes are connected to every cell in our body! Janet Goodrich's vision games Method —encouraging good vision through free movement, visualisations, emotional resolution, and relaxation is indeed related to excellent seeing.

Traditional ophthalmologists and optometrists reading this book will need the scientific data available from behavioural optometry to intellectually cross over to the promising land of Janet Goodrich's Natural Vision Improvement. For children and their parents the entry into this land will be easy.

Willemien Manschot, ophthalmologist, behavioural optometrist, the Netherlands

How to use this book

You have several ways to make this book a good friend and helpful guide:

- Read it from cover to cover.
- Use it as a referral book for subjects of interest such as switching on the whole brain or finding out why the eye must move to see clearly.
- Activate the suggested game plans suited to your child's age and vision. All vision games are in **Bold** headers in contents and text for quick reference.
- Sing. A child's first experience with music makes a permanent impression which can be called upon anytime in life for healing.

👁 Help Your Child to Perfect Eyesight

The 32 songs in this book have the power to transmute the inhumanity that we all encounter. They are designed to saturate your lifestyle and make the games easier to use. You and your children can sing and hum these tunes silently or aloud anywhere, anytime; in the car, on holidays, strolling down the hallway at school.

• Plan, record and share your experience.

Please read all chapters in the book, even when they do not apply specifically to your child. Explanations given in one chapter will refine your understanding of an item touched upon somewhere else.

The timetables at the end of activity chapters help you introduce a particular game at the right time in your child's development. Your child may be older than the suggested starting point. This does not mean that activity is irrelevant. For example, Holding Points starts at birth and continues through one's lifetime. The plus (+) sign after the month or year in the timetable means 'carry this activity forward,' regardless of age.

I use the word 'you' throughout this book. The being to whom this 'you' refers is variable. In explanatory text it refers to yourself, as parent or teacher. In descriptions of vision games, it signifies the child or children listening as you read the section aloud.

Who can benefit from using this book?

People with normal vision can use the activities in this book to increase their visual acuity. Future problems can be prevented by instilling good visual habits now.

Any child with blurred vision will benefit from using my Natural Vision Improvement programme. Guidelines are given for parents and care-givers to reverse common refractive errors. If you are the adult leading the adventure to clear sight, consider following the programme yourself. Sharing the experience is more effective than playing supervisor.

The vision improvement games are meant to become part of your family lifestyle. All the relatives can join in. Grandparents take children to the park for Cross-Crawl dancing and Magic Pencil games. Mothers relax and revive themselves while holding reflex points on their babies. Brothers and sisters with normal vision love playing Pirate Patch with a cross-eyed sibling. School teachers can calm down with massage and yawning while children palm and visualize stories read to them. The possibilities for integrating the games contained in this book into daily life are endless.

Set your mind free

- Watch. Observe. Play with the little ones.
- Learn the vision improvement games described in this book and apply them through the child's growing years.
- Enjoy a few minutes of quality time with your child each day while you both relax and play vision games together.
- Let go of the fear that your child won't be able to keep up in school or on the playground.
- Form a playgroup with friends and neighbours to do Janet's Vision Improvement activities.
- Introduce Natural Vision Improvement to your sphere of acquaintances and practitioners.
- After one or two activities have become part of your family life, introduce some new games. Take your time. Enjoy the journey!

Part One A fresh view of children's vision
Chapters 1-5

Here you will find the history of Janet's Methods, theories of cause, and suggestions for dealing with optical professionals. Chapter Four offers you a blueprint for planning and record keeping in the innovative 'Home Science' project. Share your success. Only a few parents are audacious enough to buck the system and consistently apply self-healing methods with their children. Please let us know about the obstacles to your success and how you overcome them.

The developmental stages of mental and visual growth are given in Chapter Five, helping you to decide when to introduce specific vision activities. The pace and comfort of the child is paramount at all times. Do not force, or frighten children into doing what you think they should do. Rather than saying, 'If you don't do your vision games, your eyes will get worse and you'll have to go back to glasses', you could say, 'On Saturday let's go to the park and do some Near-Far Swings on the swings.'

Celebrate small victories. A half second of straight eyes or a flash of clarity deserves applause. One incredulous father said, 'Maybe it's the change in the light' when his myopic six year old daughter named all the animals on the wall chart. She had not been able to identify them the day before. To me this little girl's ability to see the animals clearly without glasses was a normal miracle.

Part Two Keen eyesight for every child
Chapters 6-12

Learn the subtle power of reflex points and massage. Plunge into switching on the brain with Cross-Crawl, then do Swings, Sunning, Palming, and other vision games to foster good vision for yourself, your children and everyone else in your family or classroom. All the fundamental vision improvement games are explained and presented. These activities will enhance normal vision and act as a preventative to future eyestrain. They are the basis for helping children out of glasses. This section also gives you a unique way to recognise and help children with the emotions that are always tied to eyesight problems.

Part Three Specific Programs
Chapters 13-17

Use Part Three to:
- design a programme for a child who has been diagnosed with abnormal vision by an optometrist or ophthalmologist.
- find out more about the condition your child has manifested.
- learn which activities are pertinent to your child. Begin slowly and easily with the suggested games, adapting them to your child's age and your personal daily routine. One vision game a month may be perfect.
- experiment. First put the basic principles of good vision outlined in Part Two into your mind. Understand why, for example, movement is important for reversing myopia. Then you and your child can invent highly personal vision games.
- fill in the optional Home Science Programme in Chapter Five; keeping medical records and personal diary notations to document your progress with specific eye problems.

Part Four Home and school environments
Chapters 18-20

The design of diets, rooms, learning and study spaces can be crucial to the development of good vision. Modern schooling is a most unnatural process. The child sits immobilised at a desk, often in front of a flat computer screen. Eyesight and happiness both suffer. Take ideas from Part Four to educators and teachers. Urge them to provide environments that build vision rather than destroy it.

At the end of this book is a resource section to help you go shopping for toys, tools, and materials to create a colourful and inspiring environment for your child. There is a section for recommended reading on related topics. You will also find information on seminars and Instructor Training. Referral addresses for NVI teachers and other helpful practitioners are available from the Janet Goodrich Centre. You'll find the address at the back of this book.

No more glasses

The vision improvement games are generally played without glasses or contact lenses. Eyecharts, books or drawing games can be placed as close or as far away as necessary for the child's ease of seeing.

If the child's vision needs optical help, weaker than normal *Transition Glasses* can be obtained. These *T-Glasses* allow the child to function like everyone else and still give the eyes room to change for the better. Even when using Transition Glasses for school or special situations, the vision games continue. The Magic Nose Pencil and Near-Far Swings are excellent for chalkboards and computers while using weaker corrective lenses. The guidelines for obtaining Transition Glasses are in Chapter Three (pages 45-47).

Part One

A fresh view of children's vision

Chapter One

People and glasses

A brief history of glasses

The prescribing and selling of glasses is a major world industry. Most of the people involved in this industry, and their customers, take it for granted that glasses are the best thing since sliced bread. If spectacles can be a fashion item; even better. Glasses, contact lenses and a 16-second operation to shorten the myopic eyeball are helping millions of people compensate for their visual distress.

Alexander Da Spina, a monk living in the 13th century, may have put the first lenses into a frame. In the Middle Ages the wearing of glasses was a status symbol for the wealthy and intellectual segment of society. These polished stones were available from guilds and consisted of magnifiers enabling older people to read. Painters in the Renaissance depicted biblical figures wearing the latest Italian models.

Ever since ocular anaesthesia was invented in 1884 it has been possible to place thin curved lenses onto the cornea at the front of the eye. Today plastic lenses float on a layer of tears in the eyes of over 12 million Americans. However, extended wear contact lenses have inherent problems. Bacteria build-up behind the lens can cause blinding infections. Corneal cells sometimes become oxygen-starved and ulcerated. Newer contact lenses have tiny holes which oxygen molecules can penetrate.

Technologists produce better ocular aids all the time. However I still recommend that Natural Vision Improvement students do not use contact lenses. Frames are more convenient to leave off and are harder to lose. Although contacts provide more peripheral vision they deaden sensation and expressive feeling experienced through the eyes.

With glasses or contacts as the only answer, poor eyesight either stays the same or worsens. Without these optical crutches human beings would have had to acknowledge and alter the stress factors that cause vision to degenerate in the first place.

Children in glasses

Before the industrial revolution and compulsory schooling, a booming market for children's glasses did not exist like it does today. Current statistics reveal an alarming rise in the number of children with vision problems.

The American Optometric Association Task Force on Optometric Manpower in 1990 published the following estimates:

In the age group 0-4, 10 percent have refractive problems (myopia, hyperopia, astigmatism). Seven percent of these preschoolers have binocular problems.

In the age group 5-16, this number rises to 18 percent for refractive error and 8 percent for binocular problems.

By the time these children are 17-24 years of age, the numbers rise to 39 percent.

'The Catholic Digest' (November 1980) reported that 40 percent of Americans wear glasses or contact lenses for myopia, in contrast to 18 percent of the population in 1939.

This number is increasing as 'school myopia' becomes more prevalent. Hyperopia and lack of eye coordination is also of concern. Children are spending less time manipulating manual toys and more time in front of computers. This causes loss of eye-hand coordination and disturbs the act of fusion during formative years. The optical industrialists call for infant eye exams, earlier detection of amblyopia ex anopsia or 'lazy eye' and prompt treatment with glasses or eye muscle surgery.

A 12 to 20 year school experience results in distorted bodies and dulled spirits. If the school is damaging the child, why not change the school and what happens in the classroom? The Optometric Association in Adelaide, Australia is training teachers to detect vision disorders. These teachers could also be taught daily visual relaxation games. In Chinese factories and schools there is a pause each day to massage the acupuncture points related to eyesight.

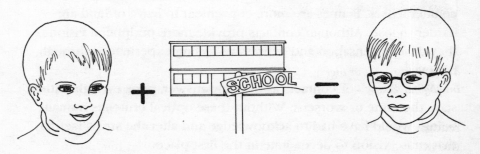

👁 Help Your Child to Perfect Eyesight

Since the early 1920s, a few scientific and medical thinkers have protested the standard response of prescribing glasses when a child or adult demonstrated visual blur. Vehemently rejected or silently ignored, the work of these people has nonetheless been sought out by thousands of ordinary folks who feel there must be a better way to see.

The beginning of the Janet Goodrich Method

I was eager to go to school. Wonderful loving teachers in the small country schools I attended smiled at me through their glasses. I sat in the square desk assigned to me, contentedly playing with my scissors and crayons. But in the midst of this joy, anxiety about succeeding and being perfect was growing inside me. By the time I was seven, I could no longer read the blackboard. When the annual school photos were taken I refused to wear my glasses. Eventually, I looked like a stranger without them.

The bridge of my nose carries the memory of metal-framed glasses. Perhaps my mother trusted none of the available optical professionals; she took me to a different one each year. The optometrists praised me for being polite, quiet, and obedient. They told my mother I had an interesting pair of eyes and that the previous optometrist had given me the wrong prescription. I was soon unable to read, play ball or get the dishes clean without my specs. My eyes became slits. I refused to look at my school photos.

At 13, I had to leave the country school where I had been the only child in my grade for seven years. I could no longer do a semester of schoolwork within the first month and spend the remaining time reading and building hay nests in the schoolyard. Playing teacher to the little kids was over. High school closed in around me like a

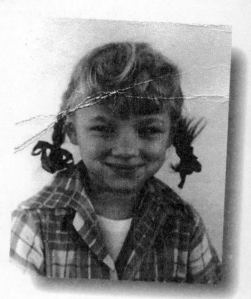

In this picture Janet is six years old. Her eyes are still soft and seeing clearly.

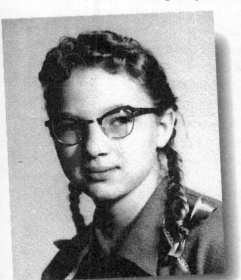

At age eleven Janet was described as a 'shy and sober, but highly intelligent child'.

straitjacket. I was too visible. I survived the internal pressure with academic achievement. Less than an A on a report card meant burning at the stake. Darell Boyd Harmon had described me perfectly in his observations of American schoolchildren. I had all of his typical symptoms: digestive problems ('All little girls have stomach-aches,' the village MD told my worried mother); aching, scratchy eyeballs behind my specs; frequent colds and pneumonia.

University was the only alternative for farm girls with high IQs. Either that or get married; or get a job with General Motors and then get married. My mind was working overtime. I decided I would never cry. By age 21 I was using -7 diopters in front of my right eye and -5 diopters in front of the left for short-sightedness and astigmatism. One eye pulled up and the other down.

At the University of Michigan hospital an ophthalmologist refused to give me contact lenses. He said my right cornea was too distorted with astigmatism. Using contacts could result in scarring. I wanted to do gymnastics and Kung Fu. The heavy frames slid down my face. A street corner optometrist in Los Angeles was happy to sell me a pair of contacts. The physical pain as I tried to get used to the contacts is etched in my mind. I lost them within three days. The pain was telling me something. I didn't know what the message was. I'd been told, 'Once a myope, always a myope'.

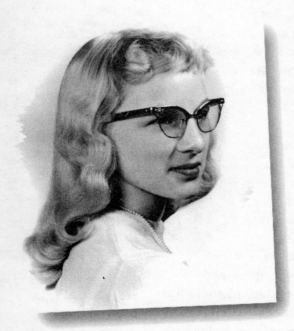

In this picture the blur-producing stare is well in place and the smile is frozen. The glasses guard the eyes and brain from perceiving too much.

Those who wanted children out of glasses

Two major teachers appeared in my life. Both these men had died before I was old enough to seek them out in person. I followed the spoor of their lives' work. The first major influence was psychiatrist and biological scientist Wilhelm Reich (1897-1957). Reich had been declared a 'medical charlatan' by a US federal judge in 1955. Doctor Reich was a student of Sigmund Freud. He parted company with that august figure, deciding that people are more afraid of pleasure than of death. Reich's ideas were violently rejected by the medical and political fraternity of his era. His ideas took seed, in spite of the burning of his inventions and publications by the US government in 1956.

👁 Help Your Child to Perfect Eyesight

Reich's ideas about child-raising are found everywhere today: natural childbirth, breast-feeding babies, giving teenagers their own rooms, open and natural sexuality, the deliberate encouragement of self-regulation and aliveness in children. Reich lived and died for these ideals.

'If I am put in jail I will die,' he stated. The judge who sentenced Reich to two years for contempt of court declared Reich's life work in biology and psychiatry fraudulent - because 'life energy does not exist.'

Suppression of natural human feelings will result in chronic muscular tension in the body. There are six large muscles outside and two smaller intricate muscles inside the eye. All perception of life is distorted by this muscular 'armouring'. In his writings, Reich described how human beings would relate to one another if they were not shielded by chronic muscular and emotional patterns:

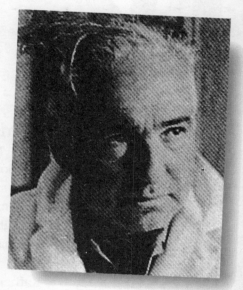

Wilhelm Reich psychiatrist

> '...they would identify with one another on the basis of the sensations of movement and rhythm. Contempt for natural movements would be foreign to them, just as they would have no comprehension of unnatural behaviour. Development would be provided for and guaranteed through the continuous production of internal energy, as in the budding of flowers... Moreover, there would be no end to the development. **Achievement would be within the framework of general biological activity; it would not be at variance with it.'**

A smog-spewing Ford carried me to Los Angeles seeking a therapy for the body, rather than for my top-heavy intellect. I wanted to be free of myopia and the constant sensation that I was not really alive. My Reichian therapist in Los Angeles took one look at my squinty eyes and said, 'Start breathing - and get rid of your glasses.' I blinked and sobbed without knowing why. Philip Curcuruto DC fostered my breathing and the melting of my body armour. I had to find a way to get rid of my glasses myself. I sought out the work of American ophthalmologist William H. Bates (1860-1931). Dr Bates published a book called 'Perfect Eyesight Without Glasses'. With his wife Emily Lierman, Bates helped hundreds of

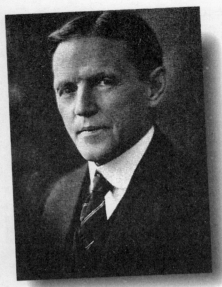

William H. Bates
ophthalmologist

children to better vision without glasses in their New York City clinic.

In the 1940s the Bates Method was made illegal in the State of New York. Although Bates' ideas are still predictably spat upon by those who sell glasses, a revised edition of his book sells steadily around the world. In the modern reprints the original copyright date of 1920 has been removed.

I have 'Better Eyesight' magazines by Bates, and his wife's book 'Stories From the Clinic'. These publications are packed with anecdotes of children improving their sight with a few visual imagery and relaxation activities. The following is an excerpt from Emily Lierman's book. Please note that she frequently uses the word 'cure'.

(Nowadays the word 'cure' is a no-no for anyone who is not a licensed medical practitioner.)

'Then a mother came to the clinic with her two little girls. Marjorie, the older, had been to us some years previously and was cured. ...The mother kept looking at me, smiling all the while. She asked: 'Don't you remember me? Don't you remember my little girl? I brought her to you and Dr Bates six years ago. She had alternate squint when she was three years old, and Dr Bates cured her without an operation.' ...Her sister Katherine, age seven years, stood by, wondering what we were going to do with her. Dr Bates examined her and said she had myopia, but not a bad case.

'I placed her ten feet from the test card and she read every letter correctly down to the 20/40 line. As I walked over to where the card was placed to assist my little patient, the mother went ahead of me and in a soft tone of voice encouraged Katherine to palm and remember the last letter of the 20/40 line of the card. Katherine did so, but she had only covered her eye for a minute when she removed her hands and opened her eyes to read again. I wanted to tell the child that she had not palmed long enough, but before I could say a word, she began to read the next line of letters as her mother pointed to each one. After each letter was read, her mother very gently told her to blink and that would help

👁 Help Your Child to Perfect Eyesight

her to see the next letter without a strain.

'When Katherine had finished reading all of the 20/30 line without a mistake, the mother did not stop, but kept right on to the next line, pointing to one letter and then another until she read all of the 20/20 line. Then the mother advised Katherine to swing her body from side to side and to notice that everything in the room seemed to move in the opposite direction. While her mother was advising her what to do, the child did the best she could to read the card. The mother smiled when she saw how amazed I was to see her improve Katherine's eyes without my help. I asked: 'Where did you learn how to do it?' She answered: 'From reading your articles in the 'Better Eyesight Magazine'. I have been a subscriber for a number of years.'

'Some months later I saw them again. Katherine's vision was 20/20 in each eye. It is interesting to report that the child was cured entirely by her mother.'

('Stories From the Clinic' by Emily Lierman, © 1926)

I found remnants of the Bates Method in Los Angeles suburbs. After her husband had been saved from blindness using Bates techniques Margaret Corbett (1890-1960) established The School of Eye Education in Los Angeles. Four vision teachers trained by Margaret Corbett were still active in LA when I arrived on the scene. One of these teachers peered at her callers from behind a locked door. She was afraid of arrest. Margaret Corbett had been tried twice for practising optometry without a licence. Aldous Huxley, author of a lovely book on the Bates method called 'The Art of Seeing', had testified at Corbett's trial. The charges against Mrs Corbett were dropped both times. State legislators refused to pass a bill prohibiting the teaching of the method. Nonetheless fresh investigations could happen at any moment. Board of Optometry officials and busybodies who didn't want to think vision training could exist outside a few optical devices, continue to harass and condemn lay practitioners of the Bates Method.

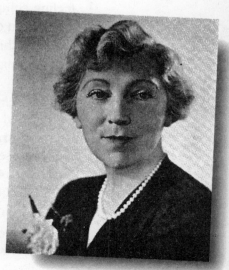

Margaret Darst Corbett

I was grateful for sessions with Hilda Reach, who had been the youngest in her Corbett training class. She revealed that Corbett teachers, who had once numbered 50 in Los Angeles alone, had disbanded their association in 1960 on the advice of a lawyer.

During the 15 years I taught my version of the Corbett-Bates method in Los Angeles, I worked with several thousand people through classes and lectures. A jittery Chicano woman came to me for a private vision session. She turned out to be an undercover agent for a government bureau. Who is this person daring to talk about eyesight without an OD after her name?

I was driving daily on the Los Angeles freeway system. I needed the help of optometrists to weaken my glasses. The fellow who assisted me did so under duress. Within two years I was able to pass my California driving test without glasses. I have been free of frames and glasses ever since. I also take exception to the use of bifocals for people over 40. I don't need correction for reading.

My life has been devoted to helping adults and children out of glasses. I regularly train people from all walks of life to do the same. There is no faculty for this at any college, although one Certified Teacher is giving Natural Vision Improvement classes at Monash University. The belief system which says 'There's no solution except glasses' has to be circumvented on a personal level.

My doctoral thesis in psychology dealt with visual armouring. It became clear to me that when Bates wrote of relaxation of the mind, he was talking about emotions. Mental stress is emotional stress. Reich's insights made it obvious that myopia in particular has a feeling component. I joined in the formation of a school that fostered expression of feelings and self-regulated learning. My children attended this school while I was teaching vision improvement classes and training as a Reichian therapist.

Honoured voices ignored

I visited the bio-medical library at UCLA with a forged pass. The books of Arnold Gesell MD, Darell Boyd Harmon, Alfred Yarbus (a Russian researcher in eye movements), and Sir Stewart Duke-Elder, (ophthalmologist to Queen Elizabeth II), fell into my hands. These men are all highly honoured names in the fields of optometry and medical science. I was greatly puzzled. Their recommendations are not put into practice.

The wholistic conclusions of Gesell, Harmon and Duke-Elder did not make it through the standardised and licensed 'refract and prescribe' habit of the optical industry. Reading the original writings of the above-mentioned gentlemen is inspiring. Arnold Gesell, pediatric ophthalmologist, observed the visual behaviour and development of 50 children from birth to age 10 at the Yale Clinic of Child Development. He writes:

> 'Human visual perception ranks with speech in complexity and passes through comparable developmental phases. Moreover, seeing is not a separate, isolated function: it is profoundly integrated with the total action system of the child: posture, manual skills and coordination, intelligence and even personality make-up. Indeed, vision is so intimately identified with the whole child that we cannot understand its economy and hygiene without investigating the whole child.'

In 1938 the Texas State Department of Health started a long range survey of children in classrooms. An inventory was made of 160 000 elementary school children; physical aspects of over 4 000 classrooms were noted. Darell Boyd Harmon published the results: 'Analysis of the data showed that at least 52 per cent of the elementary school children were leaving the school with an average of 1.8 observable preventable defects per child.' We will visit classrooms again in Chapter 20.

Alfred Yarbus researched saccadic eye movements. At the end of his book 'Eye Movements and Vision' he states, 'People who think differently also, to some extent, see differently.' The philosophical conclusions of Doctors Gesell, Harmon, Yarbus and Reich coloured the evolution of the Janet Goodrich Method. The ideas of these gentlemen are sprinkled throughout this book; they mingle congenially with the life long works of Reich, Bates, Emily Lierman-Bates and Margaret Corbett.

The techniques of John Thie DC, founder and author of 'Touch For Health' entered the picture. An evolving understanding of meridians, reflex points, and the balancing of mind and body energy seeped into NVI. Some of educator Paul Dennison's work with dyslexic children was added to the program.

While driving alone one day on the busiest freeway in the world, I heard a voice loud and clear: 'You must once again live where everything is green.' Responding to an invitation to live and teach in Australia, I loaded my three children onto an aeroplane.

During this time I wrote the book 'Natural Vision Improvement'. This was first published in Australia and is now available in the USA, Germany, France, Spain and Slovakia.

Eventually the emerald-green landing-pad of my dreams in

California appeared, nestled in the hinterland of Queensland's Sunshine Coast. Crystal Waters is a permaculture housing development devoted to care of people and care of the earth. Forty-five children live in this valley community. None of them need glasses. They attend vision play sessions for knowledge and entertainment. The Janet Goodrich Centre for Natural Vision Improvement is being built here, surrounded by thousands of young trees.

A natural way to healing

The child heals innocently. Children lie down with a fever, do not eat for a day or so - and recover their balance. Love, support and knowledge will help keep adults from interfering with this natural process. Self-love will keep us looking for causes behind symptoms and ways to support the healthy growth of the child rather than accepting the anaesthesia of glasses. Dr Duke-Elder wrote in his book 'The Practice of Refraction':

> 'Nothing is more pernicious than the routine correction of optical defects by rule-of-thumb methods. The matter is much more subtle and far-reaching. Many symptoms which are apparently caused by refractive errors or muscular anomalies would give no trouble in the ordinary course of events. They become apparent only because of ill-health or because of doing more work than the individual is capable of accomplishing with ease. A frequent instance of this is the troubles of which many children complain when commencing the routine of school life. If a rest and general tonic treatment are prescribed, these symptoms frequently disappear without any help in the form of glasses.

> '...If the latter alone are prescribed and the warning of overwork as manifested in the eyes is neglected, the glasses may provide the patient with the means whereby to struggle on until he suffers a much more serious breakdown. The adjustment of suitable lenses is not sufficient treatment in itself.'

Chapter Two

Causes of imperfect eyesight

What is eyesight?

Definitions determine actions. If seeing is a mechanical function, then a trip to the optical shop for a new pair of lenses will be satisfactory.

Honouring eyesight as a living, changing expression intimately reflecting the child's inner life will change your tactics when visual blur appears. You will hunt for the source of the problem. Glasses are given as a response to symptoms. Automatically popping glasses on children allows everyone to ignore the cause and disdain a real solution.

Who says it's faulty?

Optical practitioners prescribe glasses using two different kinds of assessment. The first is a subjective test. The child must identify letters or shapes printed in black and white on a flat card. The second part of the examination is retinoscopy, which detects refractive error in the eyeball.

The retinoscope reflects light bouncing off the retina of the eye in such a way that the practitioner can tell you if an eye is too long, as in myopia, or too short, as in hyperopia. A competent practitioner will combine these subjective and objective methods to produce an adequate prescription.

Testing vision creates blur

Does the test process itself create stress and visual blur? Reading an eyechart demands left-brain performance. Being peered at with an instrument is threatening to most children. When only the left-brain is called into play, the visual system contracts. Fear of failure and stage fright will affect the result. Through his retinoscope Dr Bates saw a child's normal eyes turn myopic. Swinging around, he glimpsed a boy from the neighbourhood staring at his patient through the window.

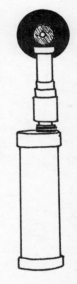

A retinoscope

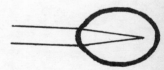

This eyeball is too long = myopia

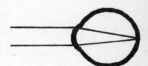

This eyeball is 'normal'

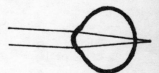

This eyeball is too short = hyperopia

The attitude and manner of the person doing the testing can also affect the results. A patient handed his previous prescription to Ken Chenery OD. It was far stronger than the refractive error that Ken had just found in the man's eyes. Ken asked what had happened during the examination. 'The optometrist was in a hurry,' was the response. Ken concluded, 'Sometimes people produce myopia to please optometrists.'

A child trying to read black and white letters or numerals is under acute pressure to give the right answers. Susan Baker at age eight resisted the test itself. 'My vision is good,' she asserted to the school nurse. She was forced to read the chart. Her mother bought a pair of glasses. Susan threw her specs into the ditch. One year later an optometrist found she had completely normal vision.

Many visual faculties are not part of the normal vision test. Colour, depth, and contrast perception are not addressed. Optical measuring cannot judge the aliveness, the sparkle, of the child's visual actions. To many doctors, personal and parental observation is 'not scientific' and doesn't count. However, only a lightly armoured adult will see aliveness in a child and remark upon its presence.

Vision fluctuates

Visual perception changes from moment to moment. I am baffled that optical professionals ignore this fact. People with normal eyesight frequently notice that fatigue, illness or an argument will blur their vision temporarily.

Within the space of one month, attorney John Rock took his five year-old son Cheney to three different ophthalmologists. All of them reported that Cheney was extremely hyperopic and needed to wear glasses all the time. Their prescriptions for Cheney varied from +2 to +5 diopters of correction. Cheney's dad did not buy glasses. He elected to take time from his hectic LA law practice to play vision improvement games on the beach with his son. Six months later, a fourth ophthalmologist examined Cheney's eyes. There was no refractive error to be found.

Theories proposed and rejected

The cause of hyperopia and astigmatism is rarely discussed in professional literature. Only recently, has lack of eye coordination and reading stress been linked to computer use.

Theories about myopia abound however, and there is little agreement about what produces it. If your practitioner has a pet theory,

👁 Help Your Child to Perfect Eyesight

please realise there are other prestigious and opposing opinions.

Myopia is inherited.

Two kinds of studies deny the inheritance theory: firstly, surveys show that identical twins are not both myopic. Secondly, the eyes of Canadian Eskimos were examined over three generations. Only five percent of the eldest generation displayed distance blur whereas 65 percent of their grandchildren were showing elongated eyeballs. The Eskimo research gave support to the 'conditions of use' theory of myopia because the grandchildren were put into missionary schools to get a proper British education.

Myopia is caused by 'condition of use'.

'Reading for too long at an early age produces a spasm in the accommodative muscle of the eye - the ciliary muscle. This chronic tension elongates the eyeball.' Optometrists who adhere to this theory think that putting minus lenses on myopic children will result in more myopia. They would rather put these children in plus magnifying lenses, and in some cases bifocals, to relax the ciliary muscle. Another proposal was to make avid young readers do something else.

In the 1930s the 'conditions of use' theory rationalised putting brilliant myopic youngsters at pottery wheels. Charles Kelley, founder of the Radix Institute in America, was a budding scientist who resented making clay pots when he wanted to read math books. Coercing this child into another occupation did not reverse his progressing myopia. With 20/400 vision at the end of high school he became a teacher of the Bates Method. He discarded his glasses while attending university and paid for his education by teaching others to do the same. No one had asked him if he wanted the pots instead of the books.

Don't discuss feelings

The Eskimo studies did not address emotional conditions. In North America indigenous children were separated from their parents and siblings, forced to speak only English, forbidden their native culture. The scientists who studied them were children of their own culture and unwilling to break its taboos. Wilhelm Reich worked long and hard to show that emotions, or life energy, moving through the organism will affect perception. When life energy is suppressed, the 'ocular segment' is frozen and perception through the eyes deadened and distorted. Post-Reichian psychologists behind thick lenses writing their PhDs on myopia felt free to ask if myopes share common emotional and personality characteristics.

Sure enough they discovered that a lot of myopes read under the blankets at night. Myopes are teachers' pets and high academic achievers. They hate to make mistakes. Near-sighted children inhibit their impulses and hide their fear. They seldom risk their humour. In contrast hyperopes throw wonderful temper tantrums. The young myope will think twice and convert her distress into a lengthy analysis.

One optometric researcher did draw a line between mental stress in school and myopia. Dr G.W. Van Alphen suggested that the pressure of doing school work starts in the higher centres of the mind-body structure. The brain shoots its 'burn-out!' message through the autonomic nerve system. The right-brain relaxation response remains turned off. This reflex normally releases stressed mechanical structures inside the eye. Therefore it is very possible that when little kids suffer over their homework the normalising mechanism for the eyes is by-passed. This can result in chronic hyperopia and myopia.

The world at large

Any change in eyesight affects the way the child feels about herself and her place in the world. The cultural factors that come to bear on a child's eyesight are of prime importance. Social ethics, comments by adults, leisure outlets and media messages all influence the child's values and choices.

An entrancing net is woven about the child in the home and on the streets. Blurred eyesight is presented both as stigma and a sign of high I.Q. The messages coming to the child are confused. Why, if the blonde princess with perfect eyesight wins the prince, should I have to wear glasses? Why, if Superman is goofy in his specs and flies through the skies hero-fashion without them, must I carry clumsy devices on my face all the time?

Americans fear three things: death, public speaking and blindness. Lack of physical vision brings no position of honour. 'Put on your glasses or you will go blind' is an excellent way to manifest what is feared. The rush to find a cure or a compensation for poor vision is understandable.

Notice how wearing glasses can be subtly rewarded. At age seven Margaret Schultz pretended to be myopic. She deliberately misread the eyechart. Her older sister was good in school and wore glasses. 'Dad loves her more. Now he will love me too.' Margaret fell into her own trap. Her eyes produced myopia to accommodate the glasses. Taking her glasses off in an NVI seminar brought back this memory of her cause.

👁 Help Your Child to Perfect Eyesight

The real cause of faulty vision

All of my experience and study tells me that visual blur is related to numerous intertwining factors.

Children lacking in self-love, for whatever reason, will seek approval from others. They contract their bodies and minds into tight knots to ensure faultless academic and social performance. Such children win the top prizes in class; and the myopic glasses.

I wish to bring the hush-hush issues of emotion, life energy and self-expression back into the picture. Working with emotional factors even mildly has helped Natural Vision Improvement students resolve life issues that have haunted them since early childhood. Dealing with feelings changes myopic and hyperopic personality patterns. Children and their companion adults can be helped tremendously with simple Emotional Healing games, such as those given in Chapter 11, that attend to their inner life.

Nutrition plays a part. Proteins, vitamins and minerals compose the structure of living eyeballs. If an essential nutrient is missing or toxic substances are entering the body, developing vision can be affected. The brain, processing input from the eyes and other senses, needs proper nutrition and plenty of oxygen. Myopes tend to consume a lot of meat and sugar. White sugar affects the body's use of chromium, important to muscular function. In Chapter 18 we will tackle the sugar challenge.

It is not normal for a child to have visual blur of any kind. **The child's environment, internal and external, causes poor vision.** Let us change that environment to the extent we are able. In chapter Four you will have a preview of developing motor and visual skills. You will be able to enter the magical, wondrous world of the child with playful vision games that fit right into the life you enjoy together.

Chapter Three

The optical industry and Natural Vision Improvement

Professional offerings

The development of the optical industry has created three main classes of professionals: ophthalmologists, optometrists and opticians. There is a fourth small group called orthoptists, who work under the supervision of ophthalmologists. It is important to distinguish between these groups and to know what each has to offer. The training and belief systems of the human beings working in these professions will affect the way your child's vision develops and the future of his eyes and mind.

The rules governing the practice of vision care varies with the country. In the USA and Australia one finds ophthalmologists and optometrists. Optometry does not exist in Germany but may do so in the future as the Common Market countries sort out the battle between already entrenched interest groups and the marketplace demands of their inhabitants. Orthoptics as a profession does not exist in many countries. Consulting the nearest library may help you to discover what services are available in your locality.

Ophthalmologists are medical doctors

Ophthalmology is a speciality branch within orthodox medicine. These medical doctors diagnose and prescribe drugs or surgery for eye diseases. They also measure eyesight for refractive errors and prescribe glasses. Opticians educated in the precision grinding of lenses fill the prescriptions. Orthoptists, predominantly women, offer children a course of eye exercises for fusion after surgery or as an adjunct to glasses.

The education of ophthalmologists is long and rigorous. In Australia students take a university degree in medicine lasting six years followed by three years of internship. Those wishing to specialise in eyes join the Registrars of Ophthalmology, a four-year course with two sets of exams. There are 768 ophthalmologists with open practices in Australia. The American Academy of Ophthalmologists lists 20 000 members with 570 of these working in paediatrics. These people are medical doctors.

'The ophthalmologist looked me straight in the eye and said, "There is absolutely nothing else you can do for your boy's eye except surgery." I didn't believe him,' the young mother explained to me on the phone. 'Simon only has a slight turn in one eye and when he is tired it gets worse. When he is happy and lively I can hardly notice the turn at all. So something must be changing.' I referred this mother to a behavioural optometrist for another opinion as she started the Natural Vision Improvement programme.

In Germany NVI teachers have taught people how to relax their eyes and improve vision in adult education schools. Annoyed by this for ten years, the ophthalmologists in that country issued an official paper titled 'Myopia Cannot be Trained Away'.

In other countries the response of medical practitioners to the Bates Method and anything similar varies from outright horror, through ignorance of the method, to complete acceptance.

Probably most ophthalmologists will say 'It can't hurt you and it can't help you. But I will be happy to monitor your progress — if you make any.'

At the other end of the rejection/acceptance spectrum stand a few medical doctors who are friends of Natural Vision Improvement. These unorthodox doctors give out eye exercises to their patients or recommend my method. They discuss nutrition with their patients. Some practise acupuncture. These rare doctors' names and addresses can be obtained from the NVI head office in Australia.

Optometrists are everywhere

Qualifying as an optometrist in Australia requires completion of a four-year degree course at an approved university, followed by board registration. Optometrists are trained to recognise eye diseases and refer any disease cases to ophthalmologists. In the USA optometrists first complete a basic science degree followed by four years of optometry school. These graduates set up a practice: you have seen their shop windows selling glasses. These folks carry OD after their names. In Asia optometrists/opticians learn the trade through apprenticeship with their relatives. They do not have formal university training; however a college of optometry has now been set up in Malaysia with 24 students.

Approximately 28 000 people practise optometry in the United States. There are currently 2 345 optometrists in Australia.

Within the group of 'straight' optometrists there are 'behavioural' or 'developmental' optometrists. In Los Angeles an optometrist checking out my vision classes informed me that behavioural optometry was 'a dying cult.'

There are 250 very alive members of this 'dying cult' in the country of Australia; between ten and 20 of them run clinics where your child can have vision training. The College of Optometrists in Vision Development in the USA lists 1 600 members, and there may be as many as 5 000 optometrists in that country who take a performance based look at their patients' visual systems. Behavioural optometrists are usually willing to weaken glasses for NVI students and to keep track of their progress.

In the 'Journal of Behavioral Optometry' Vol. 5, 1994, an article appeared, entitled 'Seeing Space - Undergoing Brain Re-programming to Reduce Myopia'. author Antonia Orfield OD described reducing her myopic glasses over a period of seven years using a variety of lifestyle improvements such as nutrition, exercise, postural training and chiropractic. Within the article is also a strong hint that putting myopic children into glasses may be counter-productive.

Seek out these optometrists to obtain weakened glasses and minimal support for your Natural Vision Improvement program. Do not expect them to agree totally with life energy concepts and leaving off glasses to allow visual and emotional change. These people like to make the changes happen with optical devices. From an information pamphlet: 'Vision therapy serves to help patients strengthen the link between vision and intelligence. Through the use of lenses and activities, it provides a patient with both development and learning experiences. The patient experiences conditions in which the old inefficient visual habits are changed into new behaviors.'

One notable exception to optometrists churning out lenses is Jacob Liberman OD who no longer puts people in glasses at all. He dares to ask his fellow optometrists to take off their glasses and contact lenses in his seminars, measuring their vision improvement after 24 hours. The results are described in his book 'Take Off Your Glasses and See'.

Even though mainstream optometry has steadily denied or

ignored the work of lay practitioners of vision improvement from the 1920s to the present, they still could not deny that the students of these teachers could read the smallest letters on the charts without glasses. The response was standardised. The oft-repeated phrases were and still are: 'You're just re-interpreting the blur. There is no real physical change.'; 'You were measured incorrectly.'; or to the over 40s, 'Your eyes just happen to be physiologically young.'

The hostility of medical doctors and optometrists to NVI and the Bates Method is based on disbelief in the usefulness of vision training and on the false assumption that Bates Method students are routinely encouraged to shun visits to eye doctors when they have disease such as glaucoma. Only the foolish would ignore a disease condition and vision training is now becoming more popular within the optical industry itself. The American Optometric Association claims that 44 percent of their 25 000 members provide some form of visual training.

It would of course be possible for NVI teachers, ophthalmologists and optometrists to work in harmony. Politics of several stripes intervene. An NVI student in Los Angeles, a dance therapist with high myopia, demonstrated great success with the programme to her ophthalmologist. The doctor then wanted to refer other patients to me, but only in secret. Disbelief in natural methods, fear of malpractice charges and peer pressure cause medical doctors to behave in their own fashion.

Times are changing. Six optometrists have taken the two month Certified Instructor Training course in the Janet Goodrich Method and some of these are conducting NVI classes for their patients.

Janet Goodrich Method teachers

Certified teachers who train with me are ordinary citizens who take a 240-hour instructors course plus practice teaching. This course includes anatomy and physiology, relaxation techniques for different kinds of functional visual blur and techniques for avoiding the wrath of medical practitioners by not pretending to have a 'cure' for anything. I insist that anyone with an eye disease seek out and remain under the care of a medical specialist. The emphasis in my method is on healing vision in a relaxed, knowledgeable and practical fashion. Teacher trainees are exposed to the psychological factors and emotional healing techniques that underpin visual styles and types. Some teachers use the emotional healing techniques and some do not. There are currently 162 certified teachers on our referral list.

Hilary Graham, certified Natural Vision Improvement teacher in Adelaide, South Australia:

> 'I usually take children from the age of six years onwards and most of them have turned or just lazy eyes. I have had great success with these children. I think that children's eye muscles are more supple and respond very quickly, round about the fifth lesson. They also love doing their vision games. One little eight year-old girl was practically blind in one eye. She didn't wear glasses as the eye specialist said that the eye was too far gone. On her fourth lesson she could read the bottom line on the close card with a patch on her good eye. Her distant vision also improved with that eye.

How to help your eye doctor give you what you want

The flaming issue for you is how to obtain support for doing a home vision programme from whichever optical professional you visit. Eye exams are needed for diagnosis and objective documentation. I personally prefer the idea of using optical devices as little as possible, but weaker lenses are often needed while eyesight is improving. The alternative to using glasses when some kind of visual aid is needed is to purchase pin-hole spectacles. Pin-hole spectacles are not prescription items, as they do not bend light. They are available in some health food stores and by mail order from us.

The parent groups at our Vision Playcamps have brought up two themes which keep them from dealing confidently with the optical professionals. The first factor is childhood training. When you step into a clinic do you hear your mother's voice saying, 'Be quiet, don't bother the busy man' or your dad's voice: 'Stop asking so many questions'?

The second factor is that both optometry and ophthalmology are exclusive clubs which inherited the Sophist style of schooling. To create such a school you first build a wall, put a sign outside the single door and make people pay a high entry fee to be able to enter. Once you've paid your money, memorised texts through long dark nights and sweated blood to serve humanity, you re-enter the 'real' world to open a clinic. Ninety-nine percent of the humans who have been through the mill to get a degree are unwilling to question the validity of what they learned in the process.

The desire on your part to blank-out and say, 'He must know what he is doing' can keep you from winning an ally inside the club. This could make a big difference in your child's vision. As a parent you have every right to question your professional friend, receiving plain English answers until you have complete understanding of your child's situation.

Blanking out and not asking the questions that haunt you in the middle of the night also allows you to lay blame on the doctor who 'should have known better.' Blaming others is the space age way of throwing options down the toilet. And don't be bamboozled by the phrase 'It's not scientific.'

The denial of the value of your own experience is made official in the statement, 'There's no scientific proof'... that vision improvement activities will improve vision problems. People who have experienced a 'flash' of clear vision without glasses, while doing one of the games in this book, know that trying to prove to a sceptic that they are seeing with crystal clarity is the surest way to fall back into the blur.

The office visit

Tell the receptionist on the phone that you intend to do home vision training with your child when you make the appointment. She can then allot extra time for your visit. Certain days and times are slower than others in the clinic. Pick a slow time to ask all your questions.

Tell the receptionist that you will be coming to interview the doctor. It is your right. Take paper and pen with you plus the following questions. The answers to these questions will form part of your Home Science records. Ask about vision in general and your child's vision in particular.

When you make the appointment use the following checklist:
- How long will my child be with the doctor?
  (Richard Kavner OD in his book 'Your Child's Vision' states that a complete vision exam for a child should take between 45 minutes and two hours.)
- Find out if the practitioner is interested in any background on the child: your pregnancy, the birth, the medical history of child and parents. These are important factors in the visual history of your child.
- Ask exactly what kinds of visual abilities the child will be tested for.
- What are the doctor's goals in treating children's vision?
- Ask for a written report in plain English, rather than scrawled medicalese. Make sure you obtain a copy of any prescriptions and that you understand what it says.

Only a few optical practitioners will state that their goal is to help children eventually get out of glasses. If you discover one of these gems, you are ahead in the game. Most practitioners will want to give the child a full 100 percent prescription that corrects his eyesight to 6/6 (20/20). If you are serious about doing my programme ask the receptionist on the phone if the doctor is **willing to give the child an under-corrected** pair of glasses. Patronization is a clear message to find a different practitioner.

If you discern that the first office is an ice cave, graciously bow out. Phone a different office and take yourself through the same process. If you feel comfortable with the service you are promised, go on to the next step.

When in the clinic be even more audacious. Ask the doctor to keep special records on your child. Is he willing to give you a discount price on regular three- or six-monthly visits so that an improvement in vision can be monitored and glasses reduced further? An optician in Singapore noticed that NVI students were rapidly dropping myopic correction. Delighted, he offered NVI students free eye exams as they improved their myopia. They paid only for their next pair of weaker lenses.

Researching surgery

Your child may be dealing with a turned eye — strabismus. Both behavioural optometrists and ophthalmologists love to treat strabismus; the first with glasses and visual training, the latter with surgery and possibly orthoptics. Studies have compared the success rate of these procedures. An article published by Nathan Flax and Robert Duckman, optometrists, shows vision training alone has a 76% cure rate.

When approaching an ophthalmic surgeon use the check list above, plus:

- What kind of anaesthesia is used for the operation?
- What are the side effects of the anaesthesia?
- What percentage of children have fusion after the operation?
- Would you kindly describe to me exactly what is done during the operation.
- Is there any follow-up check on the eyes and at what intervals?
- Do you recommend vision training instead of or after such an operation?

Some parents like to study textbooks. I was unable to obtain any information about strabismus operations from the Ophthalmology department in Brisbane. It is not given out to people who are not enrolled as medical students.

If I could not get information for researching a book on the subject, what luck would an ordinary citizen have? I tried a different tactic. One of the NVI trained optometrists in Sydney called the department of Ophthalmology at Sydney University. She was told that information about textbooks would not be given to optometrists, only to medical doctors. She was able to order the desired book for me, in her name, from her own association.

The ophthalmology textbook eventually arrived. I suggest you order these books directly from the publishers, bypassing authoritarian roadblocks.

Educate yourself to make wise decisions about your child. Be a pest and ask annoying questions in the name of love. Your child's eyes are worth it!

Obtaining and using Transition Glasses

Members of the optical industry chant, 'This child must wear his glasses or his eyes will get worse.' This threat comes out of the minds of people who do not believe that vision can be improved through natural means. You will have to skirt this mind-set. Give a megaphone to the mousey voice that whispers, 'But I wore glasses and my vision got worse.'

If you choose to trust in the innate healing power of the mind and body; if you are willing to sacrifice the values of a society which schools its children into depression and burn-out, then consider the following:

Prescription glasses lock eyes into the degree of correction. If a child relaxes for five minutes his vision will be better. When he puts on full prescription glasses, his eyeballs must serve that prescription, just as ladies used to squeeze themselves into whalebone corsets. Signs that glasses are too strong are headaches and a feeling that your eyeballs are being pulled forward out of your face. Perhaps you've experienced this when picking up a new pair of prescription spectacles, and you've been told upon questioning, 'Wear them, you will get used to it.'

Your visual system will do its best to see clearly through glass that has too high a curve in it; the curve which was determined when you were seeing at your worst under test conditions.

Eyes need room to play, to change, especially when glasses are used. NVI students often progress backwards through several pairs of Transition Glasses until they no longer need any correction.

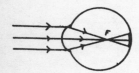

Myopic blur circle

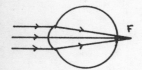

Hyperopic blur circle

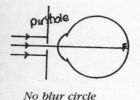

No blur circle

The guidelines for Transition Glasses have been determined by driving requirements. This level of vision is also adequate for seeing the board at school and for reading. These 'T-Glasses' allow the eyes and visual system room for improvement.

Since most children are not driving a car an important alternative for T-Glasses is to use child-sized pin-hole spectacles. Pin-holes consist of opaque plastic blanks with rows of punched holes. They are not legal for driving if there is a restriction on your driver's licence. There is no prescription involved with pin-holes and the optical industry is bypassed. Its members have used their political clout in the US and Australia to try to keep pin-holes off the market.

The pin-holes have some advantages over prescription glasses. They are inexpensive compared to the gorgeous frames sold by opticians and optometrists. They require no visits to the clinic. Vision can improve using the pin-holes until they are no longer needed.

Other pluses with the pin-holes include the fact that it is difficult to stare through them. The fly-eye effect, of looking through many holes, requires that the child keep his head moving slightly, thus releasing the back of his neck and inducing scanning rather than staring. Edging with the Magic Nose Pencil (page 96) through the pin-holes produces brilliant clarity. The marketing of pin-holes as a device that will improve eyesight by itself is misleading. Changing visual habits is what results in naturally clear vision, but the pin-holes can be a useful tool in the meantime.

However, you may not be able to find pin-holes or for some other reason your child may need to wear prescription T-glasses. In this case take the following guidelines to your practitioner in the art of prescribing and selling curved glass.

Prescription guidelines

Transition Glasses should correct the child's vision to a 'blurry' 6/12 (20/40), both eyes together for distance and close. The amount of correction in the glasses will vary with each child.

Kindly remove if possible all correction for astigmatism. If it cannot be removed completely, reduce it as much as possible. Please do not leave in the glasses correction for astigmatism less than one-half diopter. Astigmatism is one of the easiest refractive errors to erase (see Chapter 15).

No tint, anti-glare coating or UV block in the glasses please (the discussion about UV light and sunglasses for children is in Chapter Nine).

Don't use prisms to force turning eyes to straighten. Games will be done to foster the alignment and eventual fusing of the two eyes (see Chapter 16 Strabismus and Chapter 17 Fusion).

Buy plastic rather than metal frames. A metal strip running horizontally across the bridge of the nose short-circuits the governing meridian, affecting posture and brain function. The governing meridian runs from the tailbone up the spine and neck, over the top of the head and down to the upper lip.

As soon as your child is seeing better than 6/12 (20/40) through the Transition Glasses, it is time to weaken them again. This time span can vary from two weeks to six months.

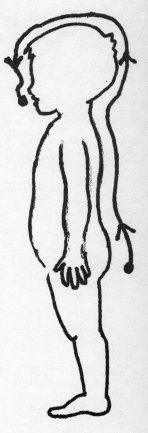

The governing meridian. The arrows show direction of life energy flow.

Chapter Four

Parent power and home science

How doctors see parents

Parents are dumb

Parents do not know and do not want to know anything about science. Therefore parents should be discouraged from thinking for themselves. If they do ask questions about vision, they should be given answers which will fit their level of ignorance and disinterest. Parents must be trained in school and through the media to obey the suggestions of authority figures. Parents must be discouraged from attempting to influence their child's poor vision in any way by telling them that such efforts would be useless or harmful. Parents should be constantly advised to make their children wear glasses and sunglasses all the time by whatever means possible.

Parents must not be asked for their opinion about the child's condition as they are not trained to detect or recognise problems. Involving the parent in the child's diagnosis could lead to wasting time and delay necessary medical intervention.

Parents must be told that their child will fall behind in school and be miserable in the classroom if steps are not taken for early detection and treatment with surgery or glasses. Everyone rightfully regrets it if a child falls behind her peers in academic achievement.

Parents will only act to the benefit of their child through fear.

Parents are wise

Given the right tools and knowledge parents are capable of helping their children to better vision within the home and family setting.

Parents are both rational and intuitive. Their love for their children when supported by appropriate ideas leads them to intelligent and effective action.

Parents are creative thinkers whose main goal for their children is health and happiness. Parents are brave beings whose hearts and minds are open to alternative and fresh avenues to healing. Parents are capable of overcoming their own fears and doubts in the face of discouragement and criticism.

Parents should be encouraged to ask questions. This helps the doctors, teachers, friends, and family arrive at the most effective approach to healing the child's vision problem.

Parents who have not yet realised all this about themselves will do so readily when given the opportunity.

Healing the parent

When you, as a parent, play vision games with your child, you will be healing both the child within yourself and your own vision. You will experience the absolute joy of discovering yourself, instead of falling into the discouragement and depression that most adults experience. The bespectacled mother who brings her child to NVI and says, 'Just fix my kid. It's too late for me' is expressing self-contempt.

Lynn Bernard, certified NVI teacher, contributed her experience:

'Meredith means "Gift from the sea/see." To truly appreciate the effectiveness of using Natural Vision Improvement techniques during pregnancy and labour one must know about the birth of Meredith's older sister. I birthed her with the very stressful mind set of "This is a hard, scary thing to do." At every decision point I took the "safe conventional route". As a result her birth was an agonizing 29 hours, every intervention made to protect the baby actually endangered her; causing further complications,. the ramifications of which are still unraveling today.

'With Meredith I had been freed of the demon of trying to please everyone else at my own expense. Because I was no longer in abject emotional pain I was able to feel with my heart what was right and see through the chicaneries of convention. I had always felt that home birth would be best for me. The Black Earth Mother that I dreamed in a Palming session during the NVI Instructor Training reappeared during Meredith's birth as my black midwife. I studied with Jeannie Parvati-Baker to train my mind to believe birth is ecstasy.

'During the pregnancy I played NVI "Painting

Pictures" many times. The night before the birth I painted a virgin forest in Virginia. The emerald green fern forest glimmered in my imagination. When the midwife arrived the next cloudy morning I was very dilated. During one contraction I was running through that virgin forest, feeling the bracken under my feet, smelling the pine, hearing the birds and finally transforming myself into a white moth. I flew into a sunbeam. From that moment on every contraction was cruising. I went into the tub. There was a cassette on called Sojourn. Later, as I examined the cassette I realized my thought patterns had followed the title of each song. I was very much in tune with my surroundings. I cried and asked my husband's forgiveness for rejecting his love so often. I was at ten centimeters in 20 minutes. This was seven hours of ecstasy. Every instant was gratifying, until I had to push. Then I clutched and had to be alone in a dark space. I remembered down to body level how wrong everything had gone at Frances' birth.

(Several hours of labour later) 'When Meredith was born the sun broke through the clouds, the sky cleared and the earth warmed. We sunned ourselves outside that afternoon.

'Even with such a tremendously beautiful birth there were complications. First Meredith refused to breathe. Then she refused to nurse. Almost immediately we found her eye was turned. We gave her a homeopathic remedy and did lots of Bird Swings together. Her eye righted itself within two weeks. Thank God Frances had no such problem. I would have totally rejected her - such had been my close-mindedness.

'I love both my daughters. It's so hard to explain this experience simply. I would love for all women to have their minds so freed that they could enjoy birth as I did or more. Some people think they can just hear or read someone saying, "Oh, my birth was ecstatic!" and assume theirs will be too. Well, it took a lot of practice to get to that point. The victims who came to me with recriminations, "Let me tell you it was no fun for me." They didn't even try to have fun. They didn't ask about

Help Your Child to Perfect Eyesight

spirituality, mind set, breathing or nutrition. I offer this story not as a boast, but so that your minds may be opened and so that you may see.'

Home Science as the new authority

The vast majority of people, including the optical industrialists, accept the mechanical response to vision because this is what they learned first. What you learned as a child and young adult in school is your truth - unless disease, disaster or sudden insight forces you to abandon the old pattern. Ordinary life does not usually pack the wallop needed to crack the initial mould; in fact it is constantly being reinforced by our social mirrors.

The mechanical response is easiest for it uses only five percent of our life energy and thumps any challengers with an iron fist. Yet life energy never dies; when thwarted it makes trouble in the eyes. Regard your child's vision development as an opportunity to directly experience life energy with its inherent up and downs. Make your own experience the highest science and top dog authority.

To gain 'proof' that your loving actions and application of natural healing do have an effect, you have to be the scientist. Science is not meant to be a cage in which ideas grow stale. True scientists observe without prejudice. They experiment with both tried and untried methods. They also document their findings and share them with others.

Your direct experience is added to the growing pool of wisdom that emphasizes what I call 'personal science' - an internal knowing that goes beyond anger or rebellion. In the past 30 years gentle birthing methods, breast-feeding and alternative health care have been growing in this way in spite of the opposition from doctors and governments. Make **your** personal science contribution. Give yourself the opportunity and the praise. Respect your own experience. Think for yourself. It's not a case of either NVI or the doctors. You can choose any combination you like, utilising the services of orthodox medical care and the actions described in this book. Bridge the gap in your own mind and come out of the illusion of isolation that parents experience when faced with an abnormal diagnosis of their child's vision.

Use the following guidelines to channel your observations, intuition, questions and answers into written form. This data will be of joy to yourself and your children when they later ask about their formative years. Twenty year-old eyes light up when age-two stories and photos come out. You will be able to stand solid in your sharing when you look back and assess the effectiveness of your loving and healing actions whether anyone else validated them or not!

Keeping a Vision Journal

I know even keeping a shopping list is difficult enough. Many of us are wounded writers after being graded in school on our fledgling compositions. How do we get ourselves to write down the precious moments of insight and small landmarks? Keep your Vision Journal simple and easily accessible. Here are a few tips:

Buy a clipboard. Hang it on a nail in the kitchen with a pen attached, or place it near the dining-table where you can sit down and write.

Buy a colourful binder and a hole-puncher.

Keep lots of plain paper in a drawer to put on your clipboard.

Keep some crayons handy for the time when the child wants to sit on your lap and draw pictures as her contribution to the journal.

Your own history
Write your history, as a mother or father.

Close your eyes and take three deep breaths.

Pretend you are talking to me or your best friend. This writing is free form. All your critics are vacationing on an island in the South Pacific. Write the following history and place it in your notebook:

My attitude towards life and my lifestyle before this child was born was...

My feeling towards children was...

The conception of this child was...

Describe the nature of the pregnancy:

a   the physical circumstances, in my body and in the environment

b   I was eating...

c   my emotional state was...

The nature of this child's birth, write about:

a   the place

b   the people

c   the mother's experience

d   the infant's state

e   Do you see any possibility of the birthing style relating to congenital eye problems?

f   Were there mechanical stresses e.g. prolonged labor, forceps delivery?

g   Were there chemical stresses? e.g. anaesthesia, smoking, toxemia. Were silver nitrate drops used? Were there toxic

substances in or around the home such as mothballs or
pesticides?

h   What time of day was this child born?

i   What were the lighting conditions at this child's birth?

j   Has one or have both of the parents used any medical drugs
such as cortisone, anti-depressants, or recreational drugs?

k   What was the medical history of the parents and grandparents?

This wonderful child

Describe your current living conditions:

a   The place, the people.

b   The child's responses.

c   Your diet, the child's diet.

d   Sleeping arrangements.

e   What's happening with eyes and vision?

f   What did you do in response to these circumstances?

g   Have you used any suggested NVI activities? If so, which ones
were you able to use? How often, approximately?

h   What changes have you noticed as a result of your own actions
to support and remedy this wonderful child's general and visual
situation? List: changes in yourself, changes in your child.

If your child is already older and a lot of history has flowed under
the bridge, may I suggest you use a timeline as shown below. Put the
key events regarding the child to the left of the line. Put your
subjective feelings and thoughts to the right of the line. For example:

Event and age	My thoughts and feelings
Bettina is born.	My cup floweth over.
At six months I notice her right eye is turning in.	I'm worried. Everyone says, 'Take her to the eye specialist'. She says, 'Come back in six months. There's nothing you can do in the meantime. She may grow out of it.'
At 18 months we go to Baby Playgroup together one morning a week.	I'm nervous about what the other parents think of me. I love being able to talk with the other mothers about the children.

Doctors' reports and prescriptions

Attach an envelope to your journal and place all doctors' reports
in the envelope. Write down your response and describe your child's

reaction to the visits to the clinic.

Add in the doctors' reports, medical treatments and recommendations, vaccination history, healing crises (illness). If you are not able to understand the doctor or optometrist's report, ask her to put it in plain English, as if you need it for a trip overseas. Make sure you understand the report enough to explain your child's condition to someone else.

The following example shows you how to read a prescription.

The number in the 'sphere' box designates the strength of the lenses for either hyperopia or myopia. A minus (-) before the number will be for myopia, a plus (+) before the number signifies a hyperopic correction. A plus lens magnifies everything you see through it, a minus lens reduces images. The cylinder and axis refer to an astigmatism correction.

	SPH (sphere)	CYL (cylinder)	AXIS
Right Eye	-2.5	-1	x15
Left Eye			

The numeral -2.5 in the right eye 'sphere' box means the child is myopic in that eye. She needs a lens with a focusing strength of two and one half diopters. Window glass has no diopters. One diopter is the amount of curve in a lens which will focus light to a point one metre away. The boxes for cylinder and axis are used only if there is astigmatism correction. This child has been given one diopter of astigmatism correction at an angle (axis) of 15 degrees. The axis is the angle of astigmatism. (Turn to Chapter 15 to understand and resolve astigmatism.) If the sphere numeral were +2.5, this child would be hyperopic.

The following pages can be photocopied. Use them to organise your Natural Vision Improvement games.

Planning Your Vision Games

Today's date _____

_____is now age _____

The doctor says _____ vision problem is

_____

_____

_____

_____

_____

_____

From chapter(s) _____ I find that we could be doing the
following activities _____

_____

_____

_____

_____

_____

_____

_____

For the last _____ month(s) we have actually been doing the
following vision games_____

_____

_____

_____

_____

_____

This is what I think and how I feel about the whole situation _____

_____

_____

_____

_____

_____

_____

What do we want to accomplish over the next three months?_____

_____

_____

_____

_____

_____

_____

These are the ways I want to go about it_____

_____

_____

_____

_____

_____

_____

_____

Send your story to:

     Janet Goodrich Centre
     12 Crystal Waters
     Maleny Queensland Australia 4552

Please send photocopies of your data pages.
Do add your feelings and thoughts. They will be read and appreciated.
Please mark the appropriate box:
❑   I wish this report to be kept confidential.
❑   Our story may be shared with others.

Signed_____

Date _____

Chapter Five

A child grows vision

What is a child?

What is your definition of a child? Are children miniature adults waiting to get big enough to work in an office? Are they extensions of parental bloodlines and egos? Or are they incarnated droplets of spirit?

Is childhood special in itself; or is it just a hallway leading to the living room? Should we stand back in awe at the metamorphosis taking place or hurry things along?

If children are adults in embryo, then keep your sights on the future adult and his place in society. The school system prepares children for adulthood in a competitive society. Young Joe will one day be supporting a family; he needs a good job. Teach him how to use a computer early. Don't let him wander by the creek. In this camp a child's vision problem is regarded solely as a blockage to performance.

This attitude toward children and education is antiquated. Management philosopher Charles Handy, author of 'The Age of Paradox', predicts that in ten years people will be holding down that 'good job' for 25, not 45 years. He encourages workers to stop thinking exclusively about careers and to develop their lives like artists' portfolios. Everyone is advised to give equal value to wages, leisure time, community service, and personal development.

Is childhood special?

Is childhood a magical time in itself? A few adults remember an ineffable glow from their childhood and the fullness of what they saw. These people look at a child and see a snowflake gleaming with uniqueness. They trust that the child contains everything he needs, to grow, heal and be self sufficient; instead of worrying about how he will carve his path.

The desire to recapture, to study and to acknowledge that there is something special about childhood must be honoured before it is too late. Samuel Silverstein, science teacher, writes:

'I believe that all children live in two worlds, both at the same time, interlocked with each other; the ordinary world that we all see as children move about in daily life, and a "hidden world" in which they are in contact with God's presence... 'a hidden world', which is available to children all the time in early childhood, but after the age of eight or so starts disappearing. Eventually it becomes mostly a "lost world"- the lost world of childhood. As adults, unless we have the ability to recall those experiences of childhood, we will have at best only hazy memories of what once occurred.'

The self-regulated child

Self-regulation allows the child to determine himself when he fits into adult schedules and demands. It also means allowing the child freedom of choice wherever possible, to change, learn and grow in his own patterns. It is freedom, but not licence.

I was proud of the fact that my baby at eight weeks was sleeping through the night. I simply could not fathom why the young mother visiting my parents was waking her baby up at night to give him his four-hourly bottle. That's one difference between the self-regulated and the other-regulated child.

There are also times when things look good to the parent but the child says, 'No' for her own reasons. When Carina was five I found a school for her that I loved. The teachers were alternative, the kids cute. There was a garden with large trees. Carina attended for two weeks. On the third Monday she refused to get off the couch and into the car. I phoned the teacher. 'Carina is playing games with you,' she said.

My respect for Carina's perception was intact. I couldn't see what was wrong with the place. She could not explain it to me. We went together to find a different school.

The child becomes the teacher in this arena. To experience the self-regulated child (I suspect one is already resident in your house), stop everything you are doing and thinking. Look at your child. Ask him what is happening, how he feels and what he would like to do about his eyesight. The response could be verbal or silent. Present him with alternatives. His choice may not please you directly but each new development of the child's abilities will show you exactly when and how to play a vision game. The following overview will alert your mind to those opportunities.

Babies are the real experts

The philosophy of treating, nurturing and helping children has been a battlefield for centuries.

Only now are the experts becoming clever enough to ask the child. In the past the observations of the mothers were seldom given any credence. This lack of interaction with the concerned parties resulted in some barbaric and unfeeling methods of dealing with children and their problems.

'There's no use dangling rattles in front of the baby's eyes,' a Melbourne ophthalmologist told a mother with a cross-eyed baby. 'There's no perception there yet.' This fellow was suffering from knowledge gap. Science has changed. By monitoring the infant's heart rate, galvanic skin response, head movements, eye movements and eager sucking, psychologists discovered that babies are sensing more than they are telling. They discovered what mothers have suspected all along. Infants are born with intelligence and a whole lot of perception. Six hour-old babies are already noting the changing expressions on mum's face and tracking triangles.

But please parents, don't run out and buy a computer for your six month-old child. Trust the pacing of the innate, the native intelligence. It comes with the package. Some of the babies being trained in the cradle to read are doing calculations in the sand at age three instead of playing with pail and shovel. It used to be that myopia began at age seven. Due to early left-brain schooling, myopia is now appearing at age four. Presenting a task before the child's motor development and brain integration is ready to perform that task may be counterproductive.

Stages of growth

The following guide is given so that you may start vision games suitable to your child's level of development.

An important hint about static timetables: if your child lags several months behind a milestone, or you feel in your heart that he is exhibiting distress, then take him to a practitioner for examination and diagnosis. But don't worry unduly if your child is tardy. The phases of childhood depicted on the timeline are averages. Many children walk at nine months. Bright-eyed, sturdy Aerro decided to walk at 20 months after becoming a virtuoso crawler. Most children are taught to read at ages six or seven. My son was more interested in swinging from the trees at that age. At 10 he proclaimed he was ready to learn reading. We spent two weeks doing Cross-Crawl, turning his reading errors into hilarious playacting. He asked for special attention at school. Within two weeks he was reading fluently. The child who regulates his own learning becomes a master.

Notice how in normal development phases children enter chaos and reorganise in a six-monthly rhythm. Negative symptoms are natural during the fall-apart phase. It's meant to be a temporary crisis. Stopping in a phase leads to chronic problems; then children get stuck in visual blur or turned eyes. Using the activities in this book may help you sail through chaos and crises.

A certified Natural Vision Improvement instructor who works with children may reside near you. If not, you may wish to take the instructor training program yourself, and/or attend one of the Parent and Child Playcamps.

Never force a child do a game. Play the game with him. If he snubs you, play the game by yourself. He will be watching out of the corner of his eye.

Infants are sensing
Birth to four months

The 'competent infant' is a new catchword in psychology. The visual system develops rapidly. These infants are no longer empty boards to be written on, nor are they 'bundles of reflexes'. Newborns are astounding in their ability to perceive visually and to respond to stimulus. Social contact and visual stimulation is most important through:

> Holding and rhythmic swinging.
> Creating an interesting visual environment (use Chapter 8).
> The rocking chair and the Bird Swing (pages 91, 100)
> Make sounds together: humming, crooning, singing, babbling, and especially yawning.
> Introduce kicking and batting toys (page 94).

At birth the baby's peripheral sighting range is 30° to the sides. At seven weeks he sees objects at 45°. By five months babies can tell the difference between a cube and a wedge.

Distance and depth perception emerge between three and six months. As soon as an infant begins to blink or reach toward an approaching object you can introduce Near-Far Swings. This is useful for babies with turned eyes (refer to Chapter 16). Do Near-Far movements with a colourful object held in your hand. Move

👁 Help Your Child to Perfect Eyesight

the object in all directions.

It is normal for an infant to alternate looking with one eye, then the other. Using both eyes together takes a big jump between 16 and 21 weeks. An infant born with a turning eye shows no acuity difference between his two eyes until he is 20 weeks old. If there is no stimulation to the brain receiving the message from the turning eye, acuity begins to drop. This fact causes some surgeons to insist that babies born with strabismus be operated on before the age of six months.

Other therapies can be used even at this early stage. Osteopathic and chiropractic consultation with a practitioner specialising in young children is available. Gentle manipulation of skull bones could repair any mechanical trauma from a difficult or forceps birth.

It is never too late to recover lost ground. Even if brain cell columns in the visual cortex have not developed properly, the body can still organize itself in a normal manner. Parents can help the rebalancing process further with regular exercises such as those found in this book, Educational Kinesiology or Kindy Gymbaroo.

Older babies explore
Eight to twelve months

Newly hatched humans are now moving from the wriggly fish stage to the independant quadruped stage. Personal status is growing. When crawling begins, a spirit of exploration appears that is insatiable. The index finger makes itself evident, pointing here and there. Touching what we see is a profound experience.

Games to play
(favouring the Phoria if need be, see Chapter 16 Strabismus)

      Peek-a-boo

      Practice walking (after he's stood by himself)

      Point to the opposite foot with the opposite hand

      Finger plays and songs

      Ball games of all sorts

      Push a ball and crawl after it

      'Let's go find something'

      Nesting boxes

      Continue mirror swings for turning eyes (page 190)

      'See it, take it, give it back'

      Bang and blink

      'Let's attach toys to strings and pull them to us'

The emergent toddler imitates

Games to play

'Get social with a group' ball games

'Monkey see, monkey does, laugh your head off'

'See what's up high, see what's down there'

Buttons sewn on things, buckles, zippers

Put large bright objects in a special vision box

'Let's take the hat on and off'

Finger plays: e.g. 'pat a cake, pat a cake...'

'Now you run and hide and I will come after you'

Sit in a circle while baby walks from lap to lap, with a hug at each stop

When walking begins, the conquering of space takes top priority. Toddlers are now interested in the fate of moving objects. The expansion of the mind is outward. Use a trip in the car or a walk, perhaps with an eyepatch on, to explore textures and things that move with appropriate verbal signals. Use the words 'look' and 'see'.

Advanced toddlers pretend

Toddlers are now learning voluntary control of muscles - potty training for example. Babbling turns into recognisable words. Manners, morals and emotions are discussed and enforced. Boundaries are established. Self-regulation does not mean abuse.

His two-sided capacities grow. Some scientists say that between the ages of three and five years the dominant side of hand, foot, eye and ear will be established. Dr. Gesell says this takes place between ages five and eight.

Games to play

Build towers and make them crash

Wrap things up in paper

Water play

Mimick sounds, gestures, faces

Play with wheels and whirlies

Putt small objects rather than big ones in the vision box

Hide-and-find games

Cross-Crawl dancing followed by other two person sports.

At age **two and one half** the child is into extremes and dualism: on and off, here and there, you and I, front and back, yes and no, asleep and awake. Intense contact with people and objects is necessary for the drive to a higher level of development. He needs 'hands on' contact with all things and people, rather than sitting

👁 Help Your Child to Perfect Eyesight

alone in front of a TV set.

The physicality of this age group means that every adult and care-giver has to get off their bottom and move. No use yelling from a distance; the exercise will do you good. Interacting in a friendly physical fashion will relax your muscles and delight the child. Tickle and massage him, instead of swatting him.

The 'tiny tyrant' may appear. This is his left-brain practice at being sure and right about his possessions and his territory. This behaviour is a protection and may become ritualised so that things are 'right there'. Crossed-eyes can appear where they weren't before. This is a perfect time to bring in directional vision games.

Three and four year-olds organise

Games to play

Matching and lotto games

Name landmarks when walking

'Let's pretend' while palming

Make things out of clay and name them

At **three and a half,** new pressures arise. Children will say, 'Don't look at me.' Earlier brain integration falls apart once more for the purpose of reorganizing on a higher level. It's necessary. Have you not noticed this in your own adult life? Grown-ups hate to fall apart. Children do not judge disintegration. They allow the intelligence of their life energy to put their body and mind back together.

While in disintegration, this child will see only one side of the story. His timing is faulty. He will drop a glass of water. Divergence may appear in the eyes and he may use the words, 'I can't see.'

Actions to take

Read a book and play Nuclear Vision games with the pictures.

Palm and pretend how you want things to be.

Act out what you imagine together. Become the lion and roar.

Make up funny names for things and people.

Use imaginary companions to sort out negative and positive emotions, then bring them together with Melting Beachballs (page 137).

At **age four,** both sides of the brain are talking to each other again. Self-confidence, expansiveness and fluidity reappear as these right-brain abilities kick in.

Games to play

Play vision games with large objects such as a metre or yard stick.

Engage in space and muscles action: skipping, climbing under chairs and tables; making a playhouse out of a table with a cloth over it.

Put on improvised dramas with animal characters.

Explore the sky, the ocean, the world while Palming.

Use round letters with Painting White on homemade eyecharts from Chapter 12.

Make large drawings with big crayons and paint.

Spend lots of time outdoors with your vision games.

Five year-olds create

This cool person is interested in fact and reality. He has things well in hand. The left-brain theme of this period makes ending things easier than starting things.

Games to play

Draw and trace with the Magic Nose Pencil (page 96).

Copy and colour (houses and homes are themes).

Start Painting White around letters, numbers and animal shapes while jumping on the trampoline (pages 146-151).

Do Feather Swings and Nuclear Vision games: in books, in the kitchen, outdoors (pages 100, 110-111).

Put letters with vertical lines on the child's eyechart.

Set up a walking board (pages 227-228).

Six year-olds question

Right-brain shifts of mood and lack of follow through reappear. The child's eyes may not want to work together. He may become ill and fatigued. Pressure about having to attend school and adhere to strict rules at the table should be eased. He may dawdle, refuse, rebel, vacillate. He may lose his place when reading. Standing up in front of the class to read aloud could become a lifetime trauma. All this is normal to the growth process. So far, the pendulum has been swinging in approximately six-month intervals through right and left-brain qualities. The intervals may become longer as the child moves into the primary school.

Games to play

Lots of Cross-Crawl dancing, yoga, stretching and body images.

Space questions: how big? how long? how far?

Oblique lines e.g. the letter K. (Letters with slanted lines can be drawn and used on the eye chart.)

Share beautiful things, sunsets, rainbows, clouds.

Vision games of pursuit-and-follow, e.g. Near-Far Swings.

Elves, fairies, and dinosaurs may appear while Palming.

Seven year-olds build

The thinker appears. He often talks to himself. He may withdraw and need a special cubby house, or a nest in the garden in a pile of mown grass. Feelings are being examined. Don't be late, and don't fail. Fantasies of packing a suitcase and leaving home arise; a map may be requested. Repetition is satisfying.

Games to play

Play ball games again. Buy a bat and softball.

Do Nuclear Vision games to find the centre of his mind and visual field (pages 106-111).

Listening is now important, so Palm with music, picking out the different instruments.

Listen to stories.

Draw and erase, then repeat the process.

Eight to 10 year-olds intellectualise

These children are competent and their brains integrated except when emotional, chemical or body stresses arise. Clubs and groups are organised. He loves to put on plays and shows; assemble toys and models. Collections of stamps and coins or stuffed animals fill shelves and drawers. Guessing what is happening from sight and hearing is enjoyed.

Games to play

'I spy' vision games, card games with eyepatches.

Make vision tests and visits to the doctor into scripts for plays.

Do lots of Painting White on self-made eyecharts
(pages 144-151).

Play games with trails, tunnels and treasure maps.

Explore the Seven Emotions with dramatic stories
(pages 132-135).

Use comics and graphic novels for tracing with the Magic Nose Pencil.

Discuss motion pictures and TV programmes while Palming.

Make eyecharts with roads and pathways leading to letters and numerals (page 144).

Part Two

Keen eyesight for every child

Chapter Six

Your child's electric body

Use reflex points to help vision

Mechanically, a reflex is an immediate involuntary response called forth by stimulating a particular area of the body. If an ant bites your toe, your eyes will immediately search for the source of the pain. Your foot will lift up by itself. This is an example of nerve reflex action. There are several kinds of reflex pathways in the human body.

In Chinese medicine, acupuncture needles are placed along meridian flow lines to ensure that *chi* (life energy) is flowing in a balanced way through the whole body. Meridians can also be stimulated by acupressure massage or by simply holding a reflex point. Meridians reflex directly to organs and glands.

If you've ever gulped down freezing cold ice-cream and felt a pain at your forehead you were over-stimulating the stomach meridian. The pain was trying to tell you something about eating ice-cold food: it damages the stomach lining.

Meridians and reflex points are part of the body's electrical system. Imagine the human body as a Christmas tree draped with chains of coloured light bulbs. The display is invisible, but it is still there. Physical malfunction or emotional distress is a signal that the lighting system needs attention.

Holding reflex points puts the plug into the electrical socket. Electrons stream through the wires, up and down. Around the tree red, green and gold areas of light radiate. OHHH, everyone sighs and feels different. Your fingers and hands are the electrical sockets full of electromagnetic energy. Contacting specific points on your child's body re-establishes and increases the flow of primal life energy.

You can use the reflex response to balance and restore life energy flow to the eyes themselves and to the visual brain, where 80 percent of vision takes place.

The effect of holding a point is immediate. I have chosen points that will be easy for you to use daily while interacting with your child. Hugging, holding, cuddling, stroking, tickling, and rocking are

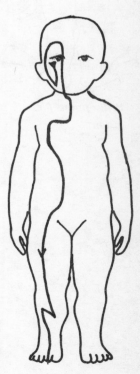

The stomach meridian is on both sides of the body.

instinctive acts. Learning the following points will give your natural caresses a healing tone.

In the 1930s, Frank Chapman, an American osteopath, discovered subtle pulses on the head which he named *neurovascular reflexes*. The rhythm of these points is unrelated to heartbeat. It may be a primitive pulsation of capillaries in the skin. Hold these points lightly; the effect is improved blood circulation to related muscles and organs. I have chosen three neurovascular points on the skull which connect directly to eyesight.

The areas to stimulate on the back are called *neurolymphatic reflexes*. These two shoulder points foster lymph flow to the eyes and related muscles. The third lower back point is used if your child has a turning eye. Nerve reflexes for the eyes are also found on the fingers and toes. This lore came from ancient India.

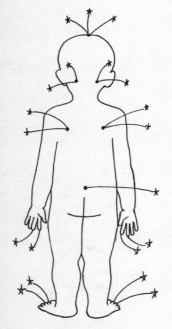

Reflex points for vision

Pre-verbal language

Emotional as well as physical messages are transmitted through the reflex points. Holding the points is like turning on a radio broadcast along with the Christmas tree lights. This broadcast is not coming through in any spoken language. It is a language which hides nothing and cannot lie.

Most adults have forgotten the unspoken language. Parents desperately ask their screaming baby, 'What's wrong with you? Do you just want attention?' By going quiet within and assuming your hunches are correct, your ability to decipher this language will sharpen.

I have named the reflex areas according to broadcasts heard while working with NVI students. If you are holding points and massaging older children, the suppressed feeling that blocked a channel may show itself. Referring to Chapter 11 will give you more ideas for unblocking rivers of sadness and volcanoes of anger.

We do not wish to deny 'negative' expressions but to be in compassion with them. For example, when holding the 'peace point' you could say out loud, 'I know you are feeling overwhelmed by life'. Once the negative is fully acknowledged and experienced, the intelligence which governs our healing process will assert itself. The 'positive' expressions come in their turn: 'I know you are capable.'

What about 'born with it'?

Babies and children are marvellously open, both physically and emotionally. You can start relating to these points from the first few days out of the womb. The less time the blockage has to establish itself,

Help Your Child to Perfect Eyesight

the less time it takes to re-activate the flow of energy through a reflex point. But start any time. You may simply have more logs to remove from the creek if the child is already 70. Even then it is the person's willingness to change that counts, not how high the log-jam is.

Even though life energy may be blocked, it is never destroyed. When it is blocked in one area, it takes itself to some other part of the body and annoys us with an ache or a twitch, and eventually with an abnormality or disease.

Life energy flows through genetic bloodlines. You inherit a landscape. Think about the flowing creek, whose source is a bottomless spring. If you dam the creek, the water will still flow even though it's not moving according to the ideal plan. It may form numerous small rivulets. It could turn your garden into a marsh. Erosion could start on the hillside. Perhaps your ancestors cut down all the trees to build houses and cooking fires. The result of that action can be inherited, not necessarily in a mathematically genetic way like haemophilia, but as a tendency or latent weakness. This helps us understand how babies can exhibit crossed eyes or come out of the womb heading in a particular direction. Head them off at the pass and re-assert the proper landscape, the proper setting for maximum recovery.

All energy blockages are attached to an experience of some kind; to a memory which may be stored unconsciously deep in the brain or in DNA. With someone who is 40 years old we might have to hold the eye points for one and a half hours before the hidden memory of almost drowning on the beach becomes conscious. On a baby of three months, holding your fingertips gently on the point for one minute at a time will re-establish the proper flow of the creek. We may wonder if the child also goes to the movies while we hold her reflex points. If she is asleep and we notice the REMs under her eyelids, we know she is dreaming. May these dreams cleanse and release family patterns, no matter how they were created or manifested.

Point Holding

The method: Place your fingertips on the points shown with a feather touch, holding them for at least as long as it takes you to hum a favorite tune or sing one of the lullabies in this chapter. These songs have been especially composed for this purpose.

Hold each point or pair of points in the **order shown.**

How often? If your baby's eyes and vision are **normal,** you can

The Wind Blows Softly

Words and Music by Donald Woodward

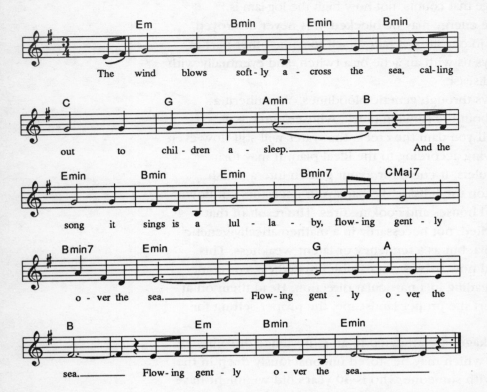

The wind blows soft-ly a-cross the sea, cal-ling out to chil-dren a-sleep. And the song it sings is a lul-la-by, flow-ing gent-ly o-ver the sea. Flow-ing gent-ly o-ver the sea. Flow-ing gent-ly o-ver the sea.

use these points occasionally. If your baby's eyes are **crossed,** or there is an indication of **abnormal vision,** hold these points every day while you are feeding or cuddling, or while the child is asleep. With older children have a 'Hold a Point Party' where you come together for a few minutes of relaxation. Older children can hold these points on themselves and on each other.

What to feel for: After you become relaxed with the idea of using your own hands for healing and after finding comfortable body positions for holding the points, you may detect a tiny pulsation through your fingers. One mother described the sensation as a 'tingling warmth' and a' tiny burst of energy'. If you don't perceive this pulse, hold the points anyway and be open to noticing it in the future.

The Peace Point

Emotion/thought:

negative   positive

'I'm overwhelmed.'   'I am at peace.'

The Peace Point is at the crown of the head. This area is called the *anterior fontanel* on a newborn. The skull bones will not have grown together completely and you can easily feel her heartbeat at this point. Move your finger to the very top of this area; your finger is a feather. Imagine the life energy rising out of this point like a

The Peace Point

👁 Help Your Child to Perfect Eyesight

fountain. The word fontanel comes from old French, meaning 'a little fountain'. We want a little fountain of energy to spring up continually from the top of the child's head.

The emotional significance of this point is peacefulness versus feeling overwhelmed. As you hold the point observe your own thoughts and body sensations. Write down your observations about feeling overwhelmed by life and its demands. See if you and the child come out of this gentle experience with a greater sense of calmness.

Loving Support Points

Emotion/thought

negative	positive
Nobody wants/loves me	Everything and everyone loves me.

At the base of the skull there are two indentations where the neck muscles attach to the skull. These are the muscles with which we nod 'yes' to life. They are powerful points for communicating love into the body. Locate these two points on yourself first. See if they are tender. Find them on your child and hold them while you both relax. You could cradle her head while she is sleeping, contacting these two points with your thumb and middle finger. If she is older and will lie down for a while, sit at her head and hold these two points with the middle fingers of both hands.

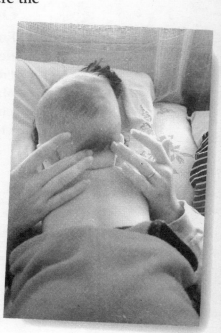

Loving Support Points

The emotional theme at these points is the question of love and being wanted. As you contact this part of the head, observe the 'theme park' of your thoughts. If this child for any reason of its own (or because it may have been picking up on your issues) is dealing with feeling unloved or unwanted, send in very clear messages aloud, in song, or in thought. Even crooning, 'You are loved. You are loved' in a singsong is releasing stress. 'The trees love you. Your Papa (Mama) loves you.' (Even if she's gone missing.) 'The birdies love you. The sky loves you'. You may end up with some hot tears in your own eyes.

Loving Support Points

Angel Wing Points

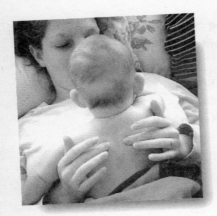

Angel wing points

Emotion/thought

negative	positive
I'm too weak	I can do anything

These two points at the corners of the shoulder blades are sore on anyone with vision problems. The divine push, the joy of creating new things turns into burdens as we grow older. The initial joy of going to school and learning turns into test stress and biting nails. This is the place from which our wings would sprout if we took ourselves lightly. Contact these points on the child by putting your two hands under the child's back from the top. Or alternately hold the points with the child on his tummy.

Ouch points

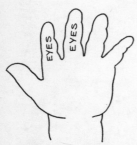

Emotion/thought

negative	positive
I'm hurting	I'm taken care of

Massage and hold these points on the fingers. When your child is older she can hold them on herself and sing this song changing the you to 'I':

Eye reflexes on fingers

You Are Loved

Words and Music by Elizabeth Ledger

Adapted by Donald Woodward

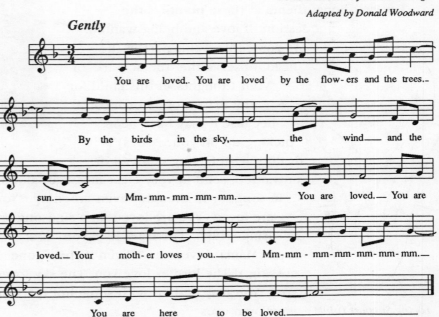

Gently

You are loved.. You are loved by the flow-ers and the trees..

By the birds in the sky, the wind and the

sun. Mm-mm-mm-mm-mm. You are loved. You are

loved. Your moth-er loves you. Mm-mm - mm-mm-mm-mm-mm.

You are here to be loved.

Help Your Child to Perfect Eyesight

Blindness points

Emotion/thought

negative	positive
I don't want to see.	Seeing is
I don't want to be seen	loving

Massage and hold these areas. If children sit cross-legged they can hold these points themselves and sing.

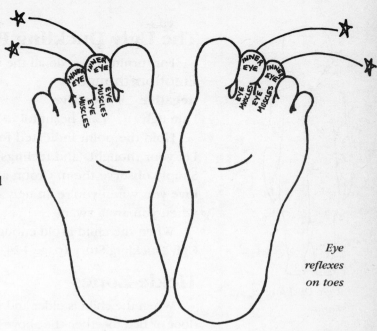

Eye reflexes on toes

The Touch Of Home

Words and Music by Donald Woodward

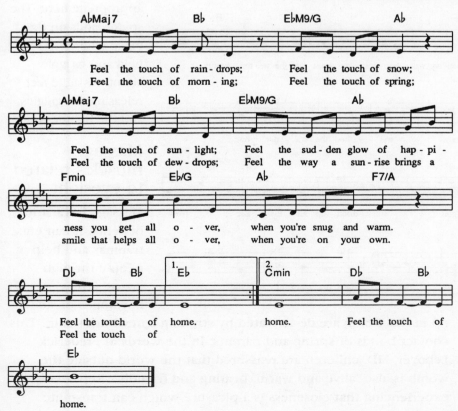

Feel the touch of rain-drops; Feel the touch of snow;
Feel the touch of morn-ing; Feel the touch of spring;

Feel the touch of sun-light; Feel the sud-den glow of hap-pi-
Feel the touch of dew-drops; Feel the way a sun-rise brings a

ness you get all o-ver, when you're snug and warm.
smile that helps all o-ver, when you're on your own.

Feel the touch of home. home. Feel the touch of
Feel the touch of

home.

The Ugly Duckling Point

For turning eyes, do all the above points plus:

Emotion/thought

negative   **positive**

I am ugly   I am beautiful

Hold the point indicated for as long as you like. Let your thoughts and feelings drift through you. Simply observe them. Croon a little tune or chant, 'I love you when you're an ugly duckling. I love you when you are a swan.'

When the child is old enough for Palming, tell the Ugly Duckling Story (page 124).

Tickle Zones

When the child is older and you are tumbling on the floor or bed together, the above points can turn into tickle spots. 'Get you right in there!' The song 'Eensie Weensy Spider' is appropriate here. The spider lands on the place where stress is held and wriggles about, his agile feet releasing the giggles and the tightness.

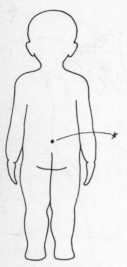

Ugly Duckling Point

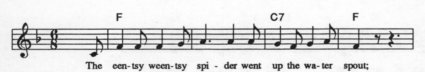

Ugly Duckling reflex area on adult spine - fifth lumbar vertebra

Eentsy Weentsy Spider

Traditional

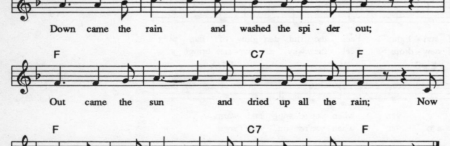

The een-tsy ween-tsy spi-der went up the wa-ter spout;

Down came the rain and washed the spi-der out;

Out came the sun and dried up all the rain; Now

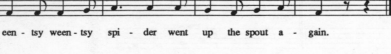

een-tsy ween-tsy spi-der went up the spout a-gain.

Massage muscles related to eyesight

Massage has many benefits. It can erase traumas and help people through crises. Stress hormones picked up in the womb are de-activated by stroking a newborn's skin. This contact bonds offspring and parents. In the words of Frederick Leboyer, MD, children are reassured that the world outside the womb is also 'alive and warm, beating and friendly'. Repeatedly experiencing that closeness is a pleasure which can transmute

👁 Help Your Child to Perfect Eyesight

difficult births or illnesses. Otherwise some of us continue to battle with life.

Make massage a family habit. After coping with fears and tears, adults also need steely shoulder muscles released. Helping others with massage and massaging oneself becomes as natural as yawning and breathing. Loosening necks and shoulders is helpful before writing a paper, or after a fatiguing performance. Through the handy aid of massage children learn that relaxation is possible under all circumstances.

Muscles are tied into the eyes through the 'Christmas tree reflex network'. Two pairs of muscles that tie directly into the visual system are the *trapezius* and the *back neck flexors*. The feet and hands may also be massaged giving special attention to the eye points on the fingers and toes.

A whole baby/child massage

With a bowl of fresh olive or vegetable oil nearby, lay baby or child down on her tummy to massage her feet for two or three minutes then proceed with the whole foot and leg. Make sure you maintain a posture that's easy on your back. Put some old towels on the dining-table or a mat on the floor. (Beds are usually too low and too soft for massage.)

Massage options:

- through clothing or undressed
- with oil from the kitchen, scented or not
- use aromatherapy (suggested fragrance: orange.)
- with music or without music

Massage your child at least once a week, more often if possible. Newborn and infant massage is recommended every day. Take every unplanned opportunity to release these muscles. It will tranquilise you as well.

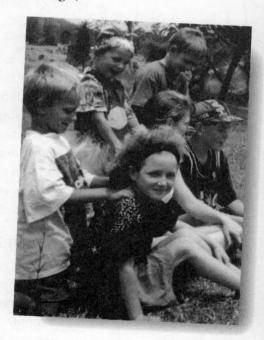

Massage for the trapezius

Since the trapezius muscles are on the back, you can either lay her on your lap or on the table on her tummy. Stroke with the flat of your hands up and down the whole back, sweeping in opposite directions with each hand. With the tips of your fingers make tiny circles up and down the spine just to the sides of the spinal processes (the little knobs where the spinal vertebrae stick out). Make a circle, lift your fingers, move to the adjacent area, make another circle. Continue in this fashion down

Everybody gets a trapezius massage.

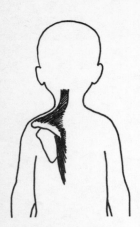

Trapezius muscle

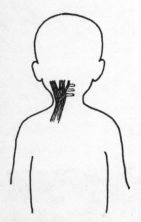

Back neck flexors

to the tailbone and up to the base of the skull. Make these small circles all along the edge of the shoulder blade. This stimulates and relaxes the areas where the trapezius and neck flexors attach to the bones. Gently knead the top of the shoulders.

Massage for neck flexors

With baby on her back, sit with her head between your legs. Reach under her neck and feel the neck muscles that run from the base of the skull down into the upper back. Using both hands together, pull up and toward you a few times. Start at the middle back and slowly proceed upwards toward the head.

Timetable for massage and point holding

For any age you could do special occasion full massages and include the eye-points. Otherwise catch your child when you can, after learning the location of reflex points and muscles.

birth to one year

Become accustomed to contacting the infant's head and body with your hands. Holding the baby in this gentle way will ease your fear about handling this tiny, delicate creature and baby will receive the language of touch which tells her she is welcome and loved within the human family. Consult massage books and have a family massage day.

two to five years

You could hold these points at bedtime while listening to the adventures of the day or playing a story on cassette. Music would be good or spontaneous story telling. Children love to become little masseuses, trading massages with you.

five to 12 years

This age group likes to learn anatomy. Painting the muscles on each other with non-toxic paint or pens will lay out the ground. Consider short massages while sitting next to each other on the couch while watching TV with Transition Glasses and Magic Nose Pencils.

No right or wrong

Are you anxious about whether you're doing things right or wrong? What's important is whether the energy is flowing. A person could do this whole method wrongly and still have successful changes take place because they did it with joy and unconditional love.

Chapter Seven

Vision is alive and well in the brain

Eyes are ruled by the brain

Seeing takes place in the child's brain, not in his eyes. Any change in eyesight reflects something happening in the brain, either a shut-down or a turn-on.

Light beams come in the front of the eye and tickle the nerve cells of the retina. The nerve cells convert light into electricity and whizz the electrical messages deep into the brain via optic nerve cables. Along the way memos are sent to other parts of the body. Ears, hands, feet, saliva glands (if a tasty meal is beaming at you) are waiting for a buzz from the head office. Sometimes the memos don't arrive or they come in late. This results in confusion, visual blur, dyslexia.

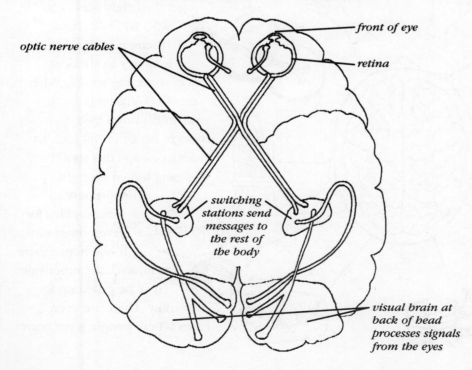

front of eye

optic nerve cables

retina

switching stations send messages to the rest of the body

visual brain at back of head processes signals from the eyes

Duelling hemispheres

There are two major sides in the brain, two hemispheres. They are joined together by a communication bridge called the corpus callosum.

The behaviour of people whose corpus callosum had been surgically severed revealed that each hemisphere of the brain is responsible for certain human behaviours.

The left hemisphere is responsible for	The right hemisphere is responsible for
• moving the right side of the body	• moving the left side of the body
• short term memory, e.g. remembering a telephone number for ten seconds	• remembering things for a long time
• talking, thinking inside the head	• imagining, visualising, making pictures in the mind
• getting all the small close-up details	• moving and grooving through space
• trying and straining to move and to see	• grasping the situation as a whole
• learning new skills	• automatic habits e.g. like riding a bike
• counting, calculating, worrying about being right or wrong.	• making music and keeping rhythm

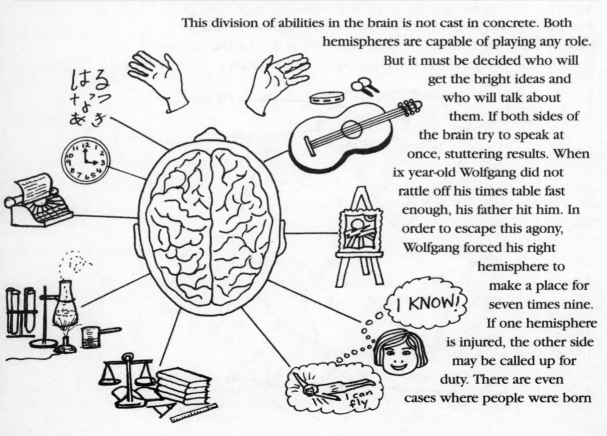

This division of abilities in the brain is not cast in concrete. Both hemispheres are capable of playing any role. But it must be decided who will get the bright ideas and who will talk about them. If both sides of the brain try to speak at once, stuttering results. When ix year-old Wolfgang did not rattle off his times table fast enough, his father hit him. In order to escape this agony, Wolfgang forced his right hemisphere to make a place for seven times nine. If one hemisphere is injured, the other side may be called up for duty. There are even cases where people were born

Help Your Child to Perfect Eyesight

with only one hemisphere and still lived normally.

When we put ourselves under prolonged physical, mental and/or emotional stress, our hemispheres stop talking to each other. We become of two minds, like a couple filing for divorce. One side says, 'Stay,' the other side says, 'Go.' One screams, 'You are not listening to me,' the other scornfully replies, 'You're acting like a child.' There may be clumsy or clever repartee but no reconciliation.

Brain battles relate directly to vision problems. The following chart shows us the attributes related to vision and which side of the brain is in action.

Left Brain 'Motor Mind'	Right Brain 'Dream Boat'
• muscle shorten, tighten	• muscles lengthen, relax
• seeing up close	• seeing in the distance
• watching the clock	• 'getting into it'
• thinking and talking	• imagining and drawing
• staying alert	• calmness of mind
• trying, straining to see	• letting everything come

It's not using one side of the brain or the other that creates chronic problems; it's **getting stuck** in one side or the other.

If muscles in and around the eyes, and the muscles of the visual reflex family, do not swing easily from relax to tense and back again, myopia, hyperopia or strabismus will result. What you can observe on the outside is a child staring and straining to see. What is not seen is the internal imbalance and everything that implies. Slap a pair of glasses on top of that inner state and the visual, emotional dysfunction remains; even though the child may perform better in the outer world.

If the child is writing words backwards, losing his place when reading, or is unable to sit still long enough to do a vision game, the two sides of the brain may be vying for the same job. More often, one side is sulking in the closet or taking off on a rocket ship. Why? Because things may be just too hard, unpleasant or just plain uninteresting around here.

The right brain will slam its door shut if it feels it is being criticised. The left brain will not sit down and add two and two if it thinks it's been abandoned. A child genius is using both sides of his brain. A genius is not a maths whiz who cannot kick a ball. Genius does both. This is the Renaissance child with no visual blur.

More compassion please

Clogged up pathways in the brain cause a breakdown in communication, failure to perform well in school, inability to express clear feelings and poor eyesight. This situation angers and frightens adults. Do you remember your own examples of this? 'She doesn't want to hear.' See if you can break the patterns of the past and find a different way to approach children, to involve them in taking care of their lives, their brain-space, with laughter and enthusiasm.

To see well, both hemispheres of the brain must be switched on and working together. Certain eye and body muscles are used to glance into the distance or at the blackboard, but when we look at a picture book those muscles must let go and let other muscles take over.

If a child is myopic, the <u>right-brain</u> is switched off for the visual system. (It could still be switched on for the gross motor level e.g. a tennis champ in glasses.)

If a child is hyperopic, the <u>left-brain</u> is switched off for the visual system. (It could still be switched on for the intellectual mind, producing a stockbroker in trifocals.)

The state of affairs in the brain will generally match itself to personality and behaviour patterns. Thus we find that scientific surveys match the above brain scenario. Myopes are perfectionists; seekers after high scholastic achievement. They will often teach themselves to read, getting a head start.

Hyperopic children are clumsy by external cultural standards. To parents and teachers these cross-eyed dreamers are cloud jockeys. Sometimes the cloud is in the middle of a cyclone.

For vision improvement we wish to get the tape-recorder-brained myope to loosen up and play more. The hyperope who takes to space games anyway needs games that will merge his dancing and hyperactivity with calmly sitting still with a caterpillar; looking at small things in a relaxed fashion so she can 'focus' on the words in her textbook.

Playing in the Hemispheres

Let us explore the land of the left brain first. In this land everyone talks: they talk numbers, they talk sense. Sometimes they talk and worry. Every moment you have to decide who's right and who's wrong. All at the same time let's talk and tighten muscles. Let's talk about who's right, but more let's talk about everything that went wrong today in detail. Do the seven times table. Tighten your

Help Your Child to Perfect Eyesight

muscles some more including the eyes, inhale and let go.

Now we are in the right part of the brain. Do you hear that humming sound? Why, that is us! Humming, buzzing and crooning, yawning, stretching, flopping, dancing, spreading our arms, bopping. Dump all the thoughts in your head into the wastebasket and be silly.

Short and long term memory game

From the cupboards and drawers find six objects that can be identified by their shape. Place the objects, without the child or children seeing them, under a towel on the table or floor. Without peeking, each child puts her hand under the towel and feels each object in turn. After taking her hand out, she tells you what the objects are. This game could be repeated at other times with different and more objects. This is left brain training.

For right brain training

Lie down on the floor together and palm your eyes by placing your cupped hands over your closed eyes. Take a trip back in time to your infancy. What is the first thing you remember? Talk about this. Trade memories. See if you can broaden the stage and see more items.

Another good way to activate long term right-brain memory is to tell the child about the cute things she did as a tiny babe or little child. Other springboards are: 'Remember your fourth birthday. What happened on that day?' 'On Christmas, when we went to visit....'

Put your brains together

It's time to blend the abilities of the two hemispheres together. Pick an ability from the left side and combine it with something from the right side.

Drawing and naming

Let's draw lots of pictures of things and give them names.

Big and little

Draw something huge. With a stick you could draw gigantic images in the sand or dirt. Make pictures on the ground with leaves. Get those images as large as possible, then reduce them to middle size. Gather twigs or pebbles and make smaller images. Go smaller still. Seeds, tiny bits of dirt. Go smaller still. How small can we get?

Sometimes a child is stubbornly stuck in a one-sided mode. Being technically correct may have won a blue ribbon in the past. In that case whimsy and colouring outside the lines may appear dangerous. If this is occurring, the best policy is to 'pace' the child. Glide alongside him for a while in the activity he has chosen. Then sneak in a laugh, a joke or a curve ball along the way. Do your best not to resist the child's resistance to immediately changing brain modes. If you do, you may get a cold shoulder.

For all eyesight problems the whole brain must get turned on, again and again and again. One of the very best ways to instantly reconcile the duelling hemispheres, the mystics with the soldiers, is with a movement called Cross-crawl.

Cross-Crawl dancing

If you move your right hand and your left foot simultaneously, both hemispheres of your brain are active. It's the same for left hand and right foot. This is the movement every human infant practises from the age of eight to twelve months by creeping. Everyone benefits from repeating the basics.

Start out on the floor. Creep under the table, between the chairs. Set some goals: roll a ball into the corner of the room and crawl over to get it. Now roll it to me. Everybody stay down at rug rat level for a time.

Move to standing. With this song practise finding right and left first.

Left and Right Song

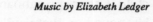

Words - Traditional
Music by Elizabeth Ledger

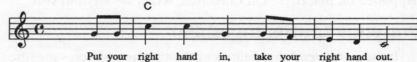

Put your right hand in, take your right hand out.

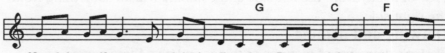

Now let's see if you can shake it all a-bout. Put your left hand in, take your

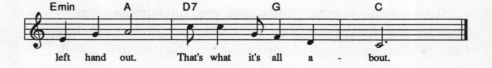

left hand out. That's what it's all a-bout.

Put your right foot in...
Put your right ear...
Put your right eye...
Put your right shoulder...

For the rest of your life

Bring your left knee up and tap it with your right hand. Bring
your right knee up and tap it with your left hand. Repeat Cross-
Crawling until you've had enough for now. This song will help you
remember it later.

Cross-Crawling

Words and Music by Elizabeth Ledger

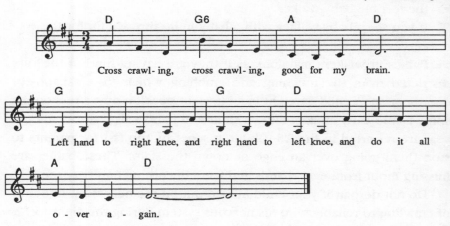

Cross crawl-ing, cross crawl-ing, good for my brain.
Left hand to right knee, and right hand to left knee, and do it all
o - ver a - gain.

Variations on the Cross-Crawl

Find objects in your visual field to Cross-Crawl with, such as the
moon, a star, a hawk, a frog, a hill, a tree, your dad, the picture on
the front of your shirt. Myopic children should Cross-Crawl at first
with objects up close, then with shapes that are farther away.
Hyperopic children do the opposite: first Cross-Crawl with a far-off
tree, then with a bush; move to a shirt button or a flower held close
to your nose.

Do a stretching Cross-Crawl dance with your favourite music.

Timetable for Cross-Crawl

birth to eight months

This group explores one side of the brain at a time. At four
months he will gaze intently at an object in his two hands held right
at his midline, but mostly he practices right or left sided movements.

eight to 12 months

Mind and body systems are ready to cross-connect the wiring.
Crawling usually begins during this time. If you think your child
would enjoy an integration boost, you can lay him on his back and
manually touch his hand to his opposite knee.

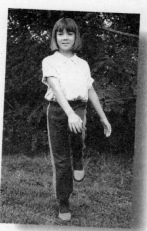

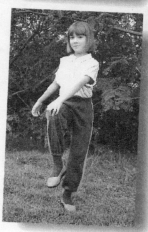

Felicity shows you the basic Cross-Crawl.

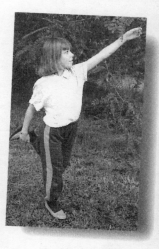

Felicity stretching in Cross-Crawl for tipuana seeds

What could interfere with the crawling practice needed to produce a brain and nervous system that will stay integrated throughout the buffets and joys of childhood?

- illness or accidents
- anxious or over-ambitious parents
- busy parents who keep their infants in playpens and/or walkers
- over-ambitious children who want to stand before they crawl
- mixed dominance (see page 87)
- the terrible baby-walker

If you see a baby-walker with a baby in it - throw a fit, for these reasons:

Babies in walkers may look as if they are having fun but they are restricted from the touching and grabbing which fosters hand-eye coordination. A child's weight in an upright position puts stress on the spine at too early an age. Fifteen thousand baby-walker accidents per year are reported in the US. Children scoot by too fast for parents to stop them going over an edge or down the stairs. These babies are missing input from eyes, hands and feet concerning empty space.

Do not despair if your child missed out on the necessary amount of crawling to reliably wire his nervous system during the eight to 12 months window. It is always possible to re-establish Cross-Crawl and repair the wiring job. Crawling is used in remedial reading programmes. Many chiropractors recommend this movement to their patients. It is standard practice in every Natural Vision Improvement class. NVI student and great-grandmother Dorothy Bryce touches opposite hand to knee when she wants to remember where she put her keys. This works for every human, including those in wheelchairs or lying in hospital beds.

one to 5 years

Let's be a cat and scratch fleas in Cross-Crawl fashion. Let's do Cross-Crawl while Dad holds out favourite toys at different positions: up high, down low, to the right, to the left, in the

Look at me in different positions while you do your Cross-Crawl.

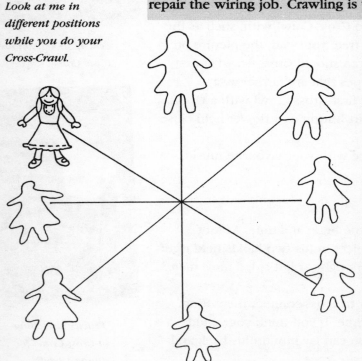

👁 Help Your Child to Perfect Eyesight

distance and finally up close. Watch that toy move to different positions while you're Cross-Crawling, so both sides of your brain are activated no matter which direction you look. Give your toy a hug. And Dad too.

five to 12 yrs

This is the age where children become self-contained. They engage in abstraction. Forming clubs is a natural to balance musing. Form a 'Lonely Brains Club' for dance parties.

Get your crayons and lots of paper. Draw the infinity sign. This sign says 'get it together' to your brain. Both hemispheres put down their weapons or get-away-cars and frolic with one another like otters under water. Put these infinity signs everywhere your eyes might fall upon them — on 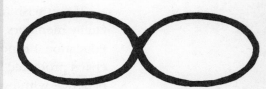 the fridge if you want to lose weight, on the computer, over your bed, inside a cupboard. If you have a task at school to perform; a test or math homework to do, always do Cross-Crawl and draw the infinity sign at the top of your page before beginning. (Cross-Crawl can even be done secretly under the desk or at the bus stop by making small movements with the fingers of one hand and the toes of the opposite foot, then repeating it on the other side.)

Use the Cross-Crawl movements as a stress-breaker with any activity, with school work, and especially in combination with all the vision improvement games coming up. If at any time you find yourselves struggling with the vision games, return to Cross-Crawl dancing.

The question of dominance

Dominance really means leadership and support. A good leader in the body receives sensory input, makes a decision, and delegates execution of his decision. Human beings take input through their five senses, then act through the motor system of the body.

'Normal' dominance would have the dominant leader brain on one side and all the executive motor agents dominant on the other side. For example, Mary is right-brain dominant. If she supports herself on her left foot to kick a ball, listens with her left ear and looks through a telescope with her left eye, then she has a normal dominance pattern. For an easy life she ought to be left-handed. Some NVI students remember being forced to use their right hand when they preferred to use their left. These people are still dealing with being punished for their natural inclinations.

'Mixed' dominance occurs when the leader brain is on one side and the ears, eyes, hands and feet are switching sides. Xavier has a dominant left brain. He uses his right hand to write and his left foot for support, and he listens to the radio with the speaker in his left ear. No wonder his nervous system gets confused and takes its own sweet time in passing memos around. Children and adults with mixed dominance need brain integration games everyday.

I have not yet found a myope or hyperope with a completely normal dominance pattern.

If you wish to find out more about dominance patterns in your family members, consult a Janet Goodrich Method Teacher or Educational Kinesiology practitioner. I feel that awareness of the chaos produced by mixed dominance grants us understanding and patience with everyone's behaviour.

Chapter Eight

Eyes must move to see
Eyes grasp the world with saccadic motion

The essential rapid flickering of eyes is called saccadic motion. In 1964 Russian biophysicist Alfred Yarbus demonstrated that if this motion stops, an 'empty field' is created within one to three seconds. 'Empty field' means no shapes, no colours; nothing is seen.

You can observe saccadic eye movements yourself. Find someone to get close to. Watch their eyeball from the side. As your specimen looks straight ahead you will see her eye making small jerky hops. This happens even when the person thinks she is 'fixing' her gaze on something.

To imagine how far your eyeball travels during an average saccadic hop, cut a pie into 10 000 pieces. Eyeballs travel across one of these pieces in one fiftieth of a second. Then they change direction.

I call this gyrating movement of the eyeballs the saccadic dance. If the saccadic dance is slowed down visual clarity is inhibited. Research saccadic eye movements of people who wear thick glasses (ask them to remove their specs); then observe people with normal vision. Long, languid saccades accompany refractive error, compared to the sparkling agile motion of normal sight.

By using the swinging and movement games in this chapter, we invite the saccadic dance to return or to remain in everyone's eyes. The dance takes place in the context of total body aliveness. Head moves, eyelids blink, lungs inflate and deflate. The whole dance hall is pulsing to the beat, even with tranquil music.

Everyone benefits from swinging and swaying. It is relaxing to body and mind.

I never use the word focus, either in this book or when teaching. The word focus is a left-brain word which connotes fixing your gaze on something. People with refractive error are already trying too hard to focus, staring and mentally working to see something. No more of that please.

Little ones do it

Eyes instinctively dance around shapes that give survival and social information.

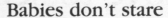

Saccadic movements around a little girl's face are depicted below left. They show how an infant's eyes would track a human face.

Babies don't stare
Observations of Aerro's mother

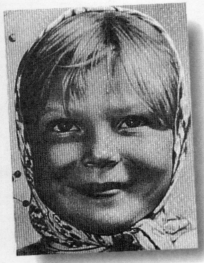

'At 13-14 days, Aerro begins to noticeably track objects. When he is swung back and forth he will strongly and sometimes very swiftly move his head to follow an image. He seems to follow in this manner most especially images with a strong light and dark contrast, such as a light bulb, or the hill-line at sunset (dark hills with light coming from behind), or changing patterns of high contrast.

'At 16 days he appears to concentrate more frequently on his parents' faces. We, his parents behave in ways to encourage these actions, by looking for images to draw his attention to, and by attempting to gain his attention and making faces for him.

'Day 18: visually he is very interested in the **motion** of his environment. When he is in input mode (i.e. having been fed and changed, awake and looking around) he becomes bored after a few minutes of lying still by himself and begins to fuss and cry. When he is picked up and carried around he immediately stops fussing and looks everywhere. When he is carried around the house he swivels his head to track various images. It now becomes apparent that he directs his attention towards **sources of light,** especially windows and door frames.

'He also enjoys lying in one's arms on his back, with his head laying back over one arm so that he is **looking at everything upside down.** So at this point he is not **recognising,** he is purely **inputting.** He will stay in this position happily for quite a while looking around. If he is also in motion, i.e. being rocked, swung, bounced on the trampoline he will turn his head back and forth a

Girl from the Volga (photo by S. Fredlyand).

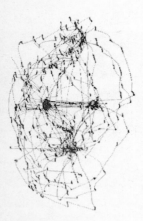

Record of eye movements during free examination of the photo with both eyes for three minutes.

Help Your Child to Perfect Eyesight

great deal, tracking images. He also enjoys music while doing this (many kinds, from Benny Goodman to Hall & Oats to Led Zeppelin) and will often fall asleep.

Note: he really enjoys motion in general, and this is usually the way to calm him, whether his eyes are open or closed. A flash thought: could this have any correlation to the necessity of movement during labour for stress relief (in labour the stress brought by pain), for him movement is soothing of various baby stresses. All humans need to move to release energy. When we are so small that we cannot really move ourselves, it seems that rocking and moving by the parents is what allows that energy release for the infant.'

Rock-a-bye my baby

One of the most important items for baby-raising is a rocking-chair. Rocking soothes mama and calms the baby. For nursing and feeding it is a must. If you bottle feed, please alternate holding the infant on right and left sides. This ensures that each eye gets stimulation during the pleasant act of suckling.

Rocking, rolling, bouncing

A voice to the child

'Inside your mama's uterus you were constantly tumbled and vibrated. Maybe your mother went for long walks; perhaps she danced or made love. Her heart was pumping close to your ears. You were born in movement and rhythms. Your care-givers instinctively pat and jounce you when you're hollering. Maybe they want some peace and quiet. It usually works. Rocking you in a chair will entertain your eyes and brain with gently moving shapes. Some babies' care-givers bought a rebounder and found that you love the tiny bounces that the two of you can make on the mini-trampoline. It puts you to sleep when you get too heavy to hold; and it pumps the lymph fluid between all the cells in your body.'

A mini-trampoline is a tool to use all one's life. It keeps people healthy and fit without jogging on a hard road. It is a lifesaver for people sitting all day in front of a computer as I am right now. The mini-tramp is two metres (six ft) away from me, flat on the floor; not propped against a wall, nor hidden in the closet. Children make a bee-line for it at Vision Playcamps.

Lymphatic pumping is good for what ails anyone. Blood is moved through the human body by the heart. Your heart will do its job even when you spend a year lying on your back. Not so the lymph system which sweeps away waste products from cells. The lymphatic network operates like canals with locks. Only movement of legs and arms opens and closes the lock. Walking while swinging your arms in Cross-Crawl fashion releases lymph locks and keeps this fluid moving. So does gentle bouncing on a well-made mini-trampoline. I say 'gentle' because too many folks think they have to start out with hard jumping. This aggravates the bladder, which first needs conditioning. Please start out on the trampoline with tiny bounces for only three minutes. You can build up from there. Hold your baby in your arms to joggle him to sleep. Aerro's favourite music for this was nuns singing Gregorian chants. When he was too big to hold, he lay on a blanket between my legs on the mini-tramp. At the top of the bounce you and baby are weightless, gravity-free for a split second.

Astronauts reported seeing trucks on highways from their perch in outer space. This superhuman acuity of vision could be attributed to weightlessness. There is no gravity drag on the eye muscles, therefore saccadic motion is faster.

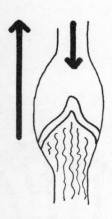

Bouncing upwards closes lymph locks

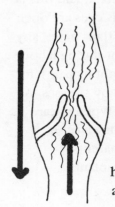

Falling downwards opens lymph locks

Dance of the Eaglet Swing

Hold baby facing outward. Turn your whole body from side to side in half a circle. Keep your shoulders aligned with your hips. This turning is done totally by your feet like a golfer's swing. Your left heel goes out as your weight shifts to your right foot. Your right foot swings out away from you as your weight shifts to your left foot. You cannot see the child's face, but be assured she is checking out all available visual shapes. This swing can also be done in front of a mirror. You and baby can check each other out as your images swing past.

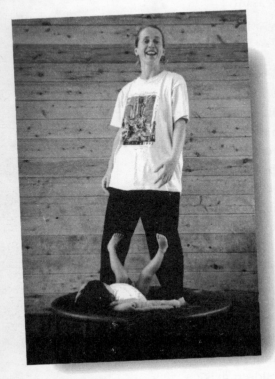

Bounce your baby to sleep

👁 Help Your Child to Perfect Eyesight

Faces

Babies are interested in other humans, especially the eyes, noses and mouths of those bigger creatures which are constantly peering into their cribs. Newborns will spend their leisure time cooing at abstract human faces. Place an image like the one below in your baby's view at a distance of approximately 22cm (7-10 in). This prepares her for relating to the new faces that will come later. Photocopy this page and/or cut out models from magazines.

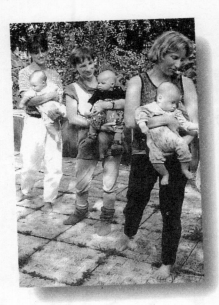

Janet and vision teachers swinging triplets

Spend time with your infant face to face. Notice how she examines you and her brothers and sisters peacefully. Watch for the saccadic dance of her eyes on your moving lips and eyes.

You could use animals also (page 94). Yarbus' research shows human eyes saccadically trace animal faces just as they do human.

Make a mobile

Eyes are attracted to edges and motion. Anything which sparkles, moves, glitters, reflects light will entertain your child's innate desire to see the world in action. Homemade mobiles can be put together in your kitchen. A newborn won't pull them into her mouth until she is about four months old. At first, place them within the 22 cm (7-10 in) range. Later you will have to move mobiles out of reach - unless they are chewable.

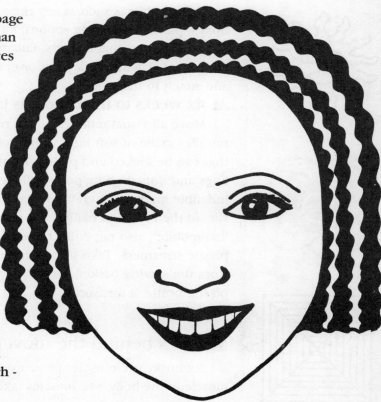

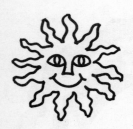

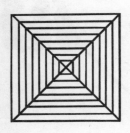

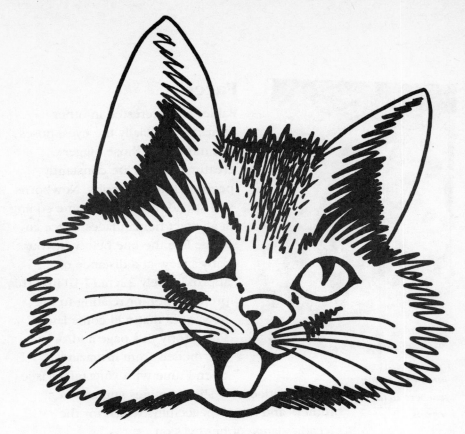

You will need coat-hangers, some string or yarn. Gather household objects such as key rings, feathers, playing cards, cereal boxes, plastic measuring spoons, kitchen sponges, costume jewelry. Attach all to the coat-hangers. Enlarge on a photocopier or draw the shapes at left with black paint or crayon. Paste them onto cardboard and attach to the mobile.

At six weeks to three months babies want to kick and bat

Move all visual mobiles out of reach and replace them with mobiles made of soft light-weight objects that can be kicked and pulled. Paint black lines and dots on ping-pong balls with indelible markers or crayons. Make two slits in the balls and hang them from the 'bat-mobile'; also rag dolls, ribbons, plastic streamers. Take some wide elastic

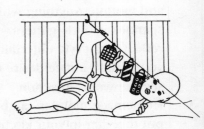

from the sewing basket; tie it tightly across the crib. Attach a plastic bottle, a measuring cup and a wooden spoon with more wide elastic.

Muscles behind the movement

Six husky eye muscles move eyeballs around. Like every other muscle in the body, eye muscles take their directives from the brain.

Help Your Child to Perfect Eyesight

Our desire is to keep the eye muscles relaxed and flexible through movement games; **not to make them work harder.**

The right brain tells muscles to relax and lengthen. The left brain tells muscles to tighten up and shorten. Proper muscle response needs both actions and both sides of the brain. The muscles moving the eyeballs work in pairs - one must pull while the

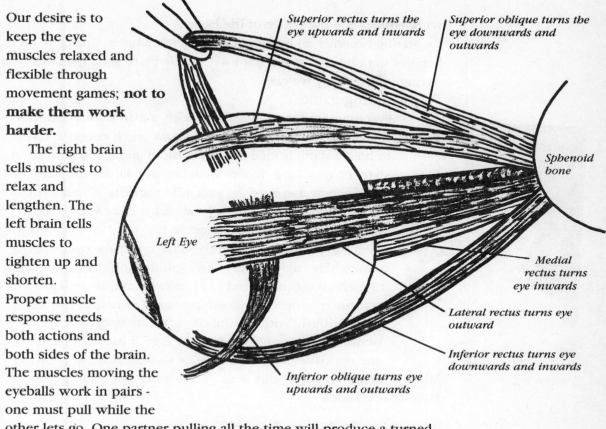

Superior rectus turns the eye upwards and inwards

Superior oblique turns the eye downwards and outwards

Sphenoid bone

Left Eye

Medial rectus turns eye inwards

Lateral rectus turns eye outward

Inferior rectus turns eye downwards and inwards

Inferior oblique turns eye upwards and outwards

other lets go. One partner pulling all the time will produce a turned eye. Two partners pulling all the time could produce hyperopia. Oblique muscles wrapped too tightly around the eyeball could create an elongated myopic eyeball. (Note: This is not a popular theory with the optical industry.)

Eye muscles

Imagine what would occur if one partner were switched off, de-activated. The other partner would have to do the whole dance by herself. She tries mighty hard but cannot win the dance marathon alone. Eventually she collapses. 'Help! We need stronger glasses.' The secret is not what most people think: 'to work at focusing'. This results in even more stress, fatigue and blur. The **stare** takes over. Anyone with functional visual blur (as opposed to blur caused by disease or accident) engages in expert **staring.** It's the glassy look on the lonesome dancer's face.

How we create blurred vision

'The cause of all imperfect sight is staring', wrote Dr William Bates. What's a stare? It's the opposite of an easy, soft, alive saccadic dance. This is why we have encouraged babies' eyes to stay loose with mobiles and the Dance of the Eaglet.

Staring becomes an unconscious body-mind habit. Changing the habit of staring helps vision improve. But first let's get a hold on staring in every way we can.

Play a staring game

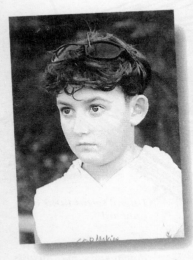

Flynn staring

Everyone produce a good hard stare; a mad stare; a sad stare. If you have normal vision, notice how much energy it takes to hold a stare. Notice that it's close to impossible for you to stare for very long. While struggling to hold a fixed stare, you may become aware of the **saccadic motion** of your eyes. If you do wear glasses, notice how easy it is for you to stare. It's an old habit, diligently practised.

To make a really good stare you have to park your eyes somewhere; tighten your jaw; stiffen shoulders and neck; tighten your tummy and hold your breath. If you can manage to worry about something, that helps tremendously with staring. Feel the stare all over your body, be aware of how much energy it uses up. Now do the opposite: Breathe. Let your shoulders d-o-w-n-n-n. Massage them. Massage your neck. Yawn a big yawn and find your Magic Nose Pencil.

The Magic Nose Pencil

It may be hiding in your pocket, or in the back of your shirt, or it could be sitting on top of your ear. Here's what the Magic Pencil looks like. Its true home is on the end of your nose.

The Magic Nose Pencil, alias the Magic Pencil, is our most important tool for breaking the stare and establishing or re-establishing a good habit of saccadic movement. This makes lots of 'nose pencilling', edging and tracing necessary for both myopes and hyperopes.

Draw everything with your Magic Nose Pencil, moving your head slightly. Eyes **automatically** seek the edges of shapes; too fast to think about it. If you hold your head still, only moving your eyeballs, you gum up the vision works. Move your whole head as you sketch with your pencil. Be more like a gesticulating Italian than a proper British professor. Relatively few Italians wear glasses. They just make gorgeous frames.

Let's do some drawing and colouring to get used to the Magic

Nose Pencil idea. Dick Bruna's picturebooks for children were praised for their simple line drawings. Edged in solid black, a little girl in bright red feeds black-edged buns to well-defined ducks.

Make your own pictures in this style on paper. Use a thick black crayon for drawing the shapes. Then fill in those shapes with brilliant colours. As you draw, keep your Magic Nose Pencil moving loosely along with the motion of your hands. When you've drawn enough Bruna-style pictures, put crayons and paper aside.

Put a pencil up to your nose. Imagine it gets long enough to reach to your dad. Put a pretend black line around him. Do it with your sister, then with the cat.

Start drawing the furniture. Drop the physical pencil, but pretend it is still there on the end of your nose. It can telescope. It gets long when you are drawing something in the distance. It shortens when you sketch something up close. Go outside with your Magic Nose Pencil, which is, of course, invisible. Draw everything around you, one shape at a time. You never have to finish a drawing, nor do you have to be careful about fine details. Loose, even sloppy drawing and edging is better than trying to be too careful about detail. This song will help you remember to edge with the Magic Nose Pencil in school, in the car, at the computer. When you talk with a friend, draw her face: eyes and nose and mouth, plus earrings and gold chains.

Trace it

Lay a picture flat on a window so that daylight shines through it. Place a sheet of plain paper over it and trace the image you want with a pen. Do lots

Magic Pencil

Music - Traditional
Words by Janet Goodrich

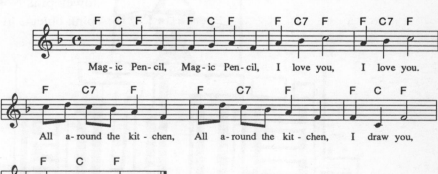

Mag-ic Pen-cil, Mag-ic Pen-cil, I love you, I love you.

All a-round the kit-chen, All a-round the kit-chen, I draw you,

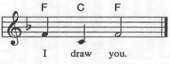

I draw you.

All around the classroom　　　　All around the music
All around the highway　　　　　All around my family
All around my bedroom　　　　　All around the people
All around the garden　　　　　　All around the foodstore

Make up any more you like!

of tracing. Then leave the pieces of paper behind. Go outside to a hillside or a patio. Pretend your tracing pencil is on the end of your nose. How many shapes can you find? Tiny green bugs, flowers, cars, your toys and stuffed animals. Line them all up and trace their shapes.

TV eyes

Parents are worried about the hours their children spend glued to the TV. I would be too. American children spend an average of six hours a day in front of the TV. Staring into a TV set keeps their eyes fixed at one distance. It dis-allows near and far practice. Hands sit idle and imagination is canned. However if the demand for TV watching is overwhelming, consider using it as a vision training tool. When my children were small, we hired a TV set each year for the month of December. You can make good use of TV for this short period: turn watching Christmas cartoons into a vision game. Trace the edges of the cartoons on the screen with your Magic Nose Pencils.

Frogs on lily pads

Lay several bath towels on the floor. These are lily pads. Sit on your lily pad and croak like a frog for a while, sketching the world around you with your Magic Nose Pencil. Crawl or hop to the next lily pad. Sketch the world again. If you have different coloured towels you could match the colour of your Magic Nose Pencil to that of each towel. Pink towel: pink Nose Pencil. Sketch all the pink objects in your visual world.

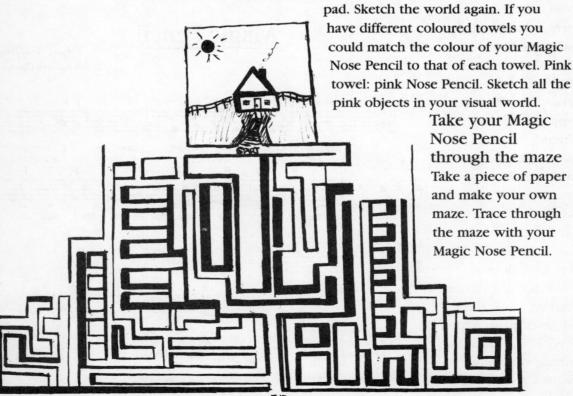

Take your Magic Nose Pencil through the maze

Take a piece of paper and make your own maze. Trace through the maze with your Magic Nose Pencil.

Join the Dots

Make your own join the dots game - join the dots with a real pencil then with your Magic Nose Pencil.

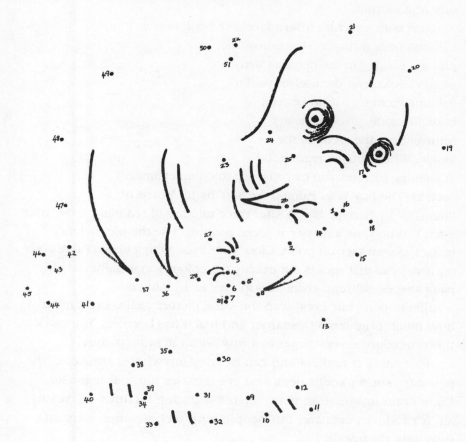

Magic Nose Paintbrush

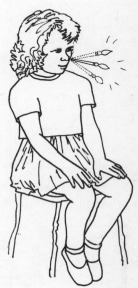

Everyone sit down comfortably. Imagine you have a **Magic Paintbrush** on the end of your nose.

It gets shorter when you paint things up close and longer when you paint things in the distance. Whatever colour you imagine in your mind will automatically come flowing out the end of your Magic Nose Paintbrush. With your eyes closed paint a red apple sitting on your hand. Feel the weight of the apple. Take a bite out of the apple. How does it taste?

Now let's paint a giant apple in the sky; a huge red spaceship-sized apple. Cover every bit of the apple spaceship with sticky red paint. This could take a while. Where does the spaceship go when you finish painting it? Paint other objects that become real.

Painting Pictures game

Painting pictures in your mind uses all parts of your brain. In addition the movement of your swishing brush produces saccadic motion.

Start with a picture from a favourite book held at a comfortable distance. Scan across the picture, soaking in the details. (Many picturebooks lend themselves well to Painting Pictures. Alison Lester's book 'Imagine' gives planetary settings from the arctic to the jungle. When you get really good at painting pictures you can advance to complex images such as 'The Boy Who Painted the Sun' by Jill Morris or 'Animalia' by Graeme Base.) After three minutes of scanning, close your eyes. You become a master at scene painting. Use the picturebook images as your take-off point. Close your eyes, with a Magic Paintbrush on your nose that squirts out exactly the colour you imagine, lavishly paint shapes, settings, characters for five to 10 minutes.

Blink open your eyes, scan the same picture again, exclaiming how much brighter, 3-D, sharper and real it has become. You can do this procedure several times in a row with the same picture.

This game is endless and can be used anywhere, any time. The painting motion keeps neck and eye muscles loose as a goose. Right-brain imagination is stimulated. Painting Pictures relaxes us all. It produces creative, fun people with technicolour, internal travelling theatres.

Bird Swing

Do the Bird Swing outdoors or indoors with music. Tune into your bird-ness. Standing with your feet firmly on the ground, swing your body in half a circle with or without baby brother. The fluffy, fantastic, flexible telescoping, Magic Feather on the end of your nose swings with you, tickling everything in sight. And everything out of sight.

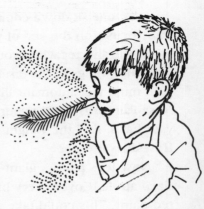

When grass gets tickled, it giggles. When trees get tickled they sigh with pleasure. When Dad gets tickled he grins.

👁 Help Your Child to Perfect Eyesight

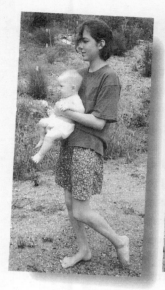
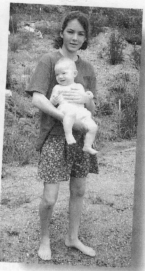
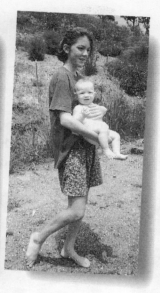

Kylie and Aerro do the Bird Swing together

When the dog gets tickled with the Magic Nose Feather, she howls. Everything responds when touched by your Magic Feather which sits on the end of your nose.

You can also tickle things secretly with your Magic Nose Feather: people in the street, the carrot in your hand just before you crunch into it. Everything comes alive when brushed with your Magic Nose Feather. As you are tickling the world with your Magic Nose Feather, you could sing this song:

I Will Tickle What I See

Music - Traditional

Words by Janet Goodrich

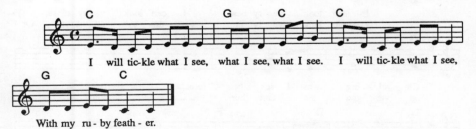

I will tic-kle what I see, what I see, what I see. I will tic-kle what I see,

With my ru - by feath - er.

2. With my bright orange feather.
3. With my yellow feather.
4. With my emerald feather.
5. With my light green feather.
6. With my sapphire feather.
7. With my indigo feather.
8. With my violet feather.

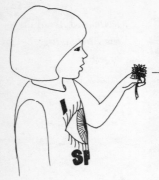

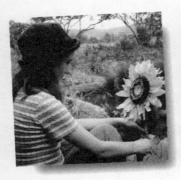

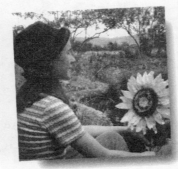

Fiona doing the Near-Far Swing with a sunflower up close and a tree in the distance

The Near-Far Swing

The Near-Far Swing is good for both myopes and hyperopes. It helps myopes bring their clear close vision outward into the distance, just like unrolling a royal carpet. Hyperopes can bring their relaxed distance vision in close with this swing.

Sit comfortably indoors or outside and find an object to hold in your hand. This could be a toy, a blade of grass, your watch. Choose an object in the distance anywhere from one metre (three ft) away to the horizon. A tree will do or a licence plate on a car or a picture on the wall.

Connect your close object and your far object with an invisible rope. Circle the close object a few times with your nose, then slide and glide, on the rope out to your distant object. Don't slide near and far with your eyeballs. Move your head, letting your nose guide your eyes.

I Can Look

Words and Music by Donald Woodward

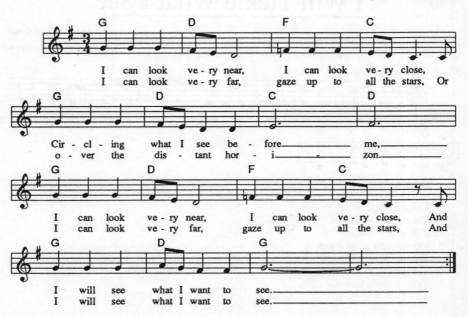

I can look ve-ry near, I can look ve-ry close,
I can look ve-ry far, gaze up to all the stars, Or

Cir-cl-ing what I see be-fore_____ me,
o-ver the dis-tant hor-i_____ zon.

I can look ve-ry near, I can look ve-ry close, And
I can look ve-ry far, gaze up to all the stars, And

I will see what I want to see._____
I will see what I want to see._____

Help Your Child to Perfect Eyesight

Circle your distant object a few times, then slide back on the rope to the object in your hand. This is a Near-Far Swing. Your rope could turn into a string of pearls, a spider's thread, a gold chain. Repeat the Near-Far Swing at least ten times on the same object; then choose another two shapes: one up close, the other in the distance.

The Near-Far Swing is fun in the house, in the kitchen, at the table. It's intriguing on a mountain top. You could create invisible lines of force making a network across the countryside.

Ball games galore

Balls are attractive to eyes. Their roundness, unpredictability and free-flowing movement irresistibly beckons interest and induces saccadic motion. Nothing moves as superbly as a ball - except perhaps the human eyeball itself. Cultivate all ball games to call forth flickery, faster-than-you-can-think-about-it saccadic eye movements.

Buy your family a collection of balls big and little, spongy ones and bouncy ones. Have a special box or basket to keep them in.

- **Roll the ball. Follow the ball with your nose.**
- **Bounce the ball. Follow the ball with your nose**
- **Play catch. Follow the ball with your nose.**

Roll The Ball

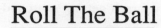

Words and Music by Donald Woodward

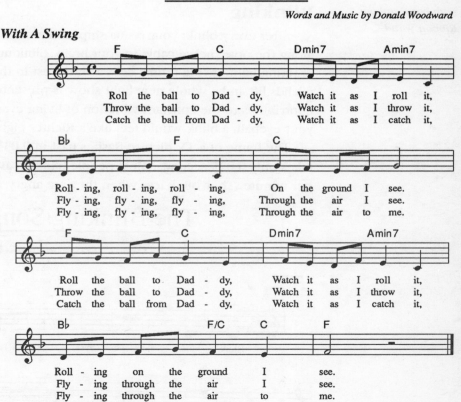

Add in anybody's name to sing and play this game with - Mommy, Michael, Katie, Jimmy, Grandma, Chinta - whoever!!

Eyes must move to see ◈

103

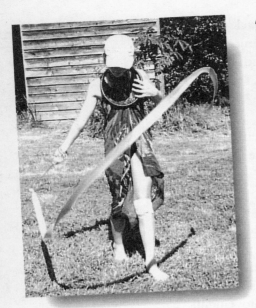

Eleanor making
an infinity sign
with her Rainbow
Ribbon Wand

The Rainbow Ribbon Wand

Make everyone a Rainbow Ribbon Wand. It brings together switching on the whole brain, movement, rhythm, total body and eye coordination.

Attach a 16 mm (1/2 in) wide ribbon which is two metres (two yds) long to a piece of dowel. The dowel could be 16-18mm (1/2 in) in diameter. The length of this stick should be about 52.4cm (20 5/8 in) long. (This length is the Egyptian cubit, a unit of measure that is meant to give strength to the body). Fasten the ribbon to the end of the stick with a thumbtack. A lovely 'lazy eight' infinity sign pattern can now be made with the Rainbow Ribbon Wand.

Turn on some music, sing or hum while making lovely patterns in the air with your Rainbow Ribbon Wand. Follow its pattern with your nose and feel yourself getting switched on.

Blinking

After every blink, your retina ships millions of bits of new data along the optic nerve cable to your brain. Blinking briefly turns off all entering light, giving retinal cells a short rest in the darkness. Then eyelids lift and a whole new light show is presented. Blinking also contributes to the constant vibration of living eyes. If you were inside your eyeball, a blink would feel like a Richter eight earthquake.

The frame of a TV picture flashes past in 0.033 seconds. A blink takes only 0.025 seconds. Most people blink an average of 20 times per minute. They blink less when they are angry, anxious or when

The Blinking Song

Music - Traditional

Words by NVI Teacher Dede Callichy

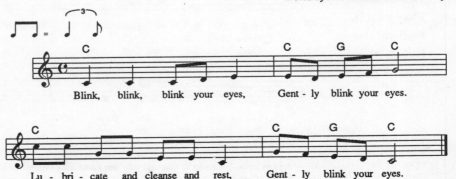

Blink, blink, blink your eyes, Gent - ly blink your eyes.

Lu - bri - cate and cleanse and rest, Gent - ly blink your eyes.

Help Your Child to Perfect Eyesight

they need to stay alert. A constant internal state of left-brain tension causes some people to hold their eyelids up until visual fatigue sets in. Then a slow effortful blink is made. These people especially need blinking practice to relax their eyelid muscles and their nerves. A bit of deep breathing and blinking helps clear everyone's vision. You can practise happy blinking with our two blinking songs.

Kibatla, Oubona * Sirourou Bell

Music - Traditional South African Song
Words by Dede Callichy

With a Swing

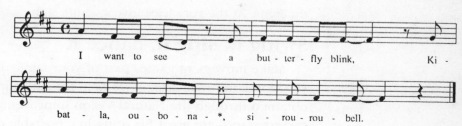

I want to see a but-ter-fly blink, Ki-
bat - la, ou-bo-na - *, si - rou-rou - bell.

* - indicates to blink, click fingers and tongue, all at the same time!

I want to see a crocodile blink, kibatla, oubona * sirourou bell.
I want to see an elephant blink, kibatla, oubona * sirourou bell.
I want to see a rhinoceros blink, kibatla, oubona * sirourou bell.

Continue changing animals.

Breathing and yawning

Eyes and brains need lots of oxygen. Deep breathing, sighing with a sound and noisy yawning provide humans, lions, tigers, hippos and lots of other creatures with necessary oxygen. Yawning also releases muscles reflexive to the visual system - trapezius and

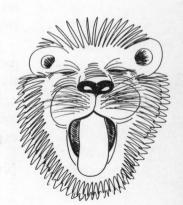

It's Cool to be a Lion

Words and Music by Bernard O'Scanaill

Slowly, In Two

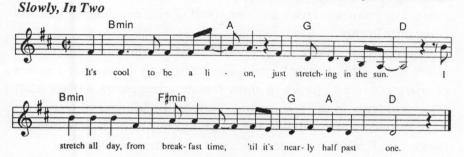

Bmin   A   G   D

It's cool to be a li - on, just stretch-ing in the sun. I

Bmin   F#min   G   A   D

stretch all day, from break-fast time, 'til it's near-ly half past one.

It's cool to be a lion,
And a lazy lion too.
I yawn all day from breakfast time,
'Til it's nearly half past two.

It's cool to be a lion,
Just swinging in a tree.
I swing all day from breakfast time,
'Til it's nearly half past three.

It's cool to be a lion,
I breathe deep when I roar.
I roar and breathe from breakfast time,
'Til it's nearly half past four.

Eyes must move to see 👁

neck flexors. It softens facial muscles and helps you change your state of mind. Your eyes give themselves a bath by yawning. Vision brightens up as if you had washed the world as well as your eyes. Make a sound with your exhalation. This could be a loud roar with the lions. At the very least give a gentle sigh.

Swing it, sing it, dance it

Make movement games part of your family lifestyle. Adult vision will improve also. More help for adults in glasses can be obtained through the Natural Vision Improvement book. My cassette tapes are great for using in a portable cassette player while walking or driving. Sing Eyes Songs walking to school; at the dinner table; in the bath.

Timetable for movement

birth to one+ years

Set up mobiles. Swing, rock and gently bounce babies until they are just too heavy to hold.

one to five+ years

This is the time for dancing, looking near and far, and ball games galore. Blink, stretch, yawn.

five to 12+years

Introduce the Magic Nose Pencil, Feather and Paintbrush. Do the Near-Far Swing, Yawning, and Painting Pictures Game. Make everyone a Rainbow Ribbon Wand.

Nuclear Vision

Your mind, eyes, and brain have a common characteristic. They use the concepts of foreground and background in the same way a landscape artist does. However a painting on the wall is flat and static. The paintings created in our visual system are dimensional and constantly in flux.

Interest determines foreground. One day, while crossing the street in LA I was nearly hit by a car. I distinctly remember a series of sharp coloured images - a shiny fender, a red panel, a black glob of tar suddenly in the foreground. The sky, buildings and trees were in that moment dulled in colour and blurred. They became background. My feet pushed me away from the car without consulting my left-brain. I thumped on the car and yelled, 'Are you blind?'. The driver wasn't blind; he just wasn't interested in pedestrians. 'Sorry, I didn't see you.' It was a good thing I had not

👁 Help Your Child to Perfect Eyesight

been staring. I avoided injury because important bits of light were fed into my *fovea centralis* and visual brain in a 100th of a second. And the memo reached my feet in time.

Quickness of eye, mind, and brain is slowed down by all the stress factors that interfere with brain integration; with the passage of messages from one hemisphere to the other, and to the hands and feet. If the light beams from that front fender had not entered my fovea I could still be limping. If I had been in a myopic stare, or worrying about being hit by a car, the lightning-rapid foveal messages could have been delayed.

People with refractive error have lowered foveal or central vision. My name for this ability to see clearly what you are interested in is Nuclear Vision. This 'sharp-shooter' eyesight can be recovered and honed with Nuclear Vision games. Nuclear Vision is **not concentration and a tight focus** where all peripheral shapes are blanked out. Sharp central vision needs peripheral, background blur for its very existence. It is a paradox. If a person with refractive error fights the blur and tries harder to see, she will create more blur. Clarity needs blur just as the distinct foreground of a painting needs a hazy background, just as day needs night. Surprisingly, heightening the blur makes sharp central vision reappear. The following Nuclear Vision games will help everyone restore excellent central vision.

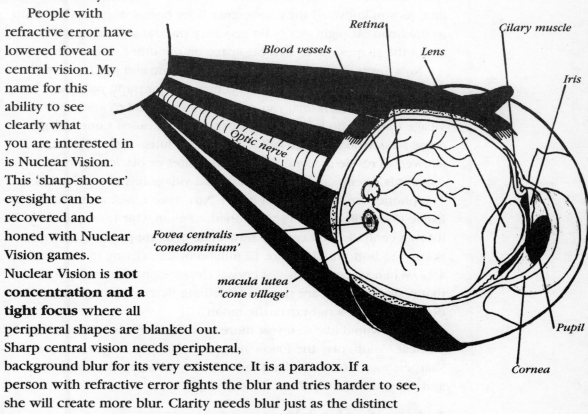

A trip to Fovea Centralis

Everyone lie down and close your eyes. Let's hop into a boat and blow magic shrinkage dust over it. It gets smaller and smaller. It gets so small we can float right through the pupil of our eyes, through the lenses of our eyes, back to a spreading, curved, red wall called the retina.

Notice the rich orange colour of this healthy retina. See crimson-red rivers ladened with oxygen-rich blood. These streams feed our *cone* and *rod* cells with nutrients. Larger blue rivers are carrying garbage away from the cells. Out here in the countryside (the outer areas of our retina) rods that see black and white and cones that see colour and details live side by side. This is blur country. Everyone here is laid back and not too hyped up about making things clear. In fact our rod cells still use old-fashioned party-line phones — six to a line. As you know, all the phone lines from retinal nerve cells end up in the brain. At night our brain gets very unclear and vague messages about the shapes out in that big space on the other side of our pupil.

Now I want to show you our greatest pride and joy. If you will kindly take a direct line from the centre of your pupil right back to the centre of your retina, you will find, I am proud to announce, a village that was built here many years ago. It's called Cone Village. Some folks who dig Latin call it the macula lutea. Only cones are allowed to reside in Cone Village. No whites or blacks allowed: only coloureds. Every single cone cell in that village has its own phone. The phones are red, blue and green. Now take a look at that high rise inside Cone Village. That's the Conedominium. Our Latin visitors call it fovea centralis. You can see how cone cells are packed in there bottom to bottom. There are 12 million of them living in that small area. When you get a flash of crystal clear vision, the cone phones in that conedominium are ringing something fierce. Your colour and detail vision goes right over the moon.

If you would like to invest more time in the thrills and ecstasy of Nuclear Vision, play the following games. Nuclear Vision games will sharpen your already brilliant mind, help you conquer school work and get your arrow right in the bull's-eye.

Intensify the blur

It's strange. The way to clear vision is not to try to see your object of interest more clearly, but to intensify the blurry surroundings. You do this by talking to them. When you are circling a red petunia, ask all the other flowers to be less bright, less alive than your petunia. Corbett teachers had children do this with two candles. Hold two lighted candles about 26 cm (one ft) apart. Swing your attention from one candle to the other. Pause at one candle and tell the other candle to be blurred. Keep on doing this as you gradually bring the two candles together. Penlights or coloured pencils work just as well as candles.

The Nuclear Junk Box

Fill a box with all kinds of things: bottle tops, feathers, keys, marbles, screws, pet pebbles. Dump the contents out on the table, floor, or ground. Circle each item with your nose, thereby moving your whole head. That's your foreground object. Tell all the other pieces of junk to 'blur off'. They constitute your background. Emphasize the blurriness of the background. You'll notice the object of your attention becomes clearer.

Counting games

There are zillions of seashells strewn on the beach. When you start to count them you have to single out one seashell at a time. The light

When I Count

Words by Janet Goodrich
Music by Donald Woodward

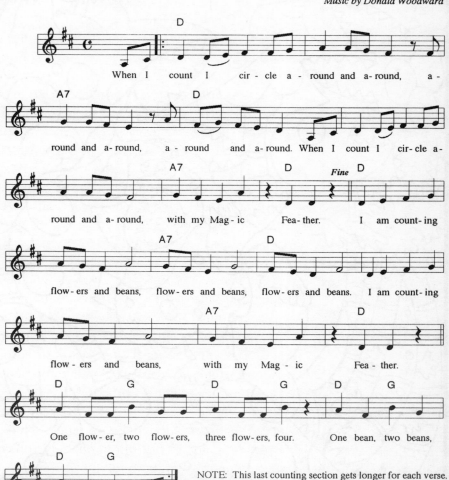

NOTE: This last counting section gets longer for each verse. After the last verse, return to the beginning, then finish at *Fine*

I am counting leaves on the trees, leaves on the trees, leaves on the trees...
One leaf, two leaves, three leaves, four leaves, five.
When I count I circle around...

I am counting bees and birds, bees and birds, bees and birds...
One bee, two bees, three bees, four bees, five bees, six.
One bird, two birds, three birds, four birds, five birds, six birds, seven.
When I count I circle around...

I am counting clouds in the sky, cars on the road, clouds in the sky...
One cloud, two clouds, three clouds, four clouds, five clouds, six clouds, seven clouds, eight.
One car, two cars, three cars, four cars, five cars, six cars, seven cars, eight cars, nine cars, ten!
When I count I circle around...

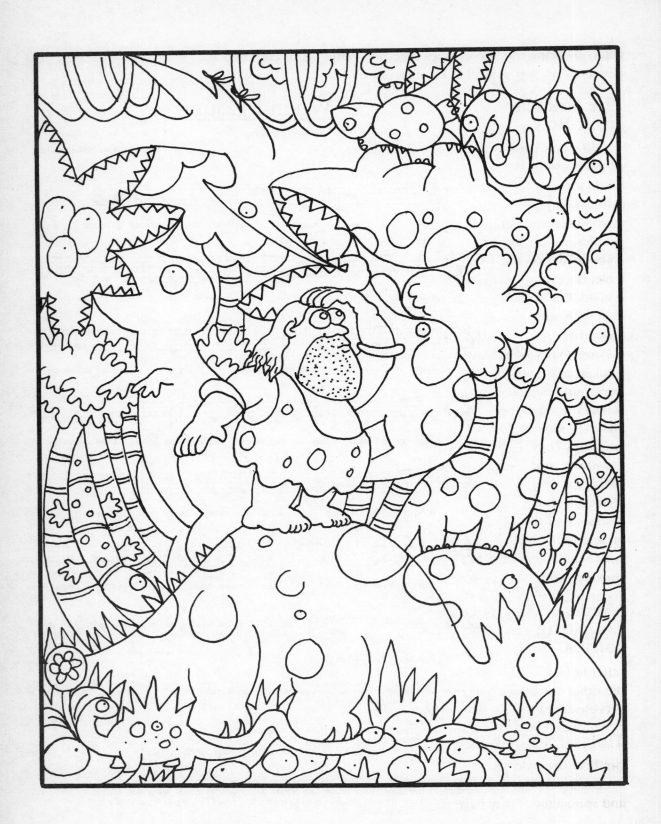

👁 Help Your Child to Perfect Eyesight

beams reflected off the mass of seashells is the background. The shell you assign a numeral to is, in that moment, your foreground. Its lightbeams ought to ring the phones in your Conedominiums. On the beach you would do this by circling a seashell with your nose and crying out, 'One seashell'; then 'Two seashells'; 'Three seashells'. Continue to count as high as you would like, always circling and being aware that the other seashells are more blurred than the one you are circling. How many different objects can you count in this way? Do your counting with a song (page 109). It's music for your right-brain and numbers for your left-brain.

Hidden Pictures

Hidden Pictures games hone your ability to keep one shape constant in your mental and visual foreground, even as you move through a varied background (which could be a jungle where only the sharp-eyed stay relaxed and alive). On page 110, Con the Caveman is looking for his lost pets. Help him find them. This game requires at least two players. The Finder Player closes her eyes while the Describing Player picks out an animal from the picture and gives its name to the Finder. The Finder paints this animal with his Magic Nose Paintbrush for a few seconds.

The Finder opens her eyes while retaining the image of the animal in the back of her mind. The Finder scans the prehistoric landscape with a nose feather until the creature imagined comes alive and leaps out of the background. The Finder must then celebrate in an appropriate manner to the applause of the Describer. I'm so much more interested in the process of this game than whether you get the right answer that I don't even give you the answers in the back of this book.

Nuclear vision on eyecharts

Put an eyechart on the wall where you can see the top three rows on the chart clearly (pages 144-148). Circle one letter and tell all the other letters to 'blur off'. Move to another letter or shape and tell all the other shapes to 'blur off'. Notice that the shape you are circling gets clearer, all by itself.

Timetable for Nuclear Vision games

birth to five years

During this period a natural interchange of sounds, songs, words and spontaneous play pave the way to Nuclear Vision.

five to 12+ years

The concept of 'blurring off' peripheral shapes can now be introduced. Use candles and junk box activities to get the idea and feeling of Nuclear Vision. Then use your Magic Nose Paint Brushes to circle and count shapes in picturebooks and on eyecharts. It's fair to use Nuclear Vision when taking eye tests.

Chapter Nine

Mad about sunlight

Are sunglasses good for kids?

It had been raining in Germany for ten days. When the grey drizzle finally stopped, I stood on the veranda of the seminar house and welcomed the sun as it peeked over the lofty oak trees. Diamond droplets glittered on every leaf. I closed my eyes, drinking in warm, cleansing sunlight. I was alone that morning on the veranda until a participant in a yoga course walked past. 'Beautiful!' she exclaimed as she noticed how much I was enjoying the morning glow. As she exited the veranda she turned and shot back at me, 'But the sun is dangerous'.

When I mention that Germans who speak English can take the instructor's course in Australia, their eyes glaze over with fear. 'But what about the hole in the ozone right above Australia?' they ask. In this country government campaigns convince people they must slap on sunscreens and pop on sunglasses as soon as they step out the door. Many parents buy infant sunglasses and tie them on the baby's head. There is a rumour that sunglasses may become part of required school uniform in schools in Brisbane.

UV-anxiety sells shiploads of Taiwanese sunglasses and tons of chemical soups for the skin. The general public rarely hears about the beneficial aspects of UV light. It is true that too much UV light can burn the skin and the eyes. Too much water, heat, or vitamin A can also be harmful. There is another side to the story. Take notice when media reports and scientific irrationality overwhelm your intuition and inquiring nature. Here is what John Ott, author of 'Health and Light', says about UV light and life on planet Earth:

> 'Another school of thought believes that while too much ultraviolet is definitely harmful, normal amounts of these forms of energy found in nature may be essential to the healthy growth and development of both plants and animals. In addition to all the new products designed to protect people from the so-called harmful effects of any trace amount of ultraviolet, come

others that are designed to let through the natural ultraviolet in sunlight and add the normal amount of ultraviolet that is lacking in artificial light sources.'

At St. Paul's Catholic School in Brisbane the Bolle company supplied free sunglasses to primary grade children in a behaviour modification experiment to convince children to wear sunglasses all the time. Australian ophthalmologists believe that exposure to UV light causes *cataracts* (deposit of opaque substance in the lens of the eye) and *pterygiums* (a fatty yellow tissue growth on the cornea). If, they reason, children can be persuaded to wear sunglasses all their lives, when they are 60 they will not have cataracts and pterygiums. On the phone one medical expert told me his evidence was not conclusive. He is unable to do the 40- or 50-year follow-up study which would prove that lifelong use of sunglasses will prevent eye disease; but 'It's enough.' When I questioned him about the research showing some UV stimulation is essential to general health, he replied, 'I'm not convinced that UV light through the eyes is important.'

Other ophthalmologists believe cataracts and pterygiums are caused by faulty nutrition. Dr Gary Price-Todd states that eye diseases can be prevented and healed with nutritional supplementation.

For every scientific paper printed in ophthalmological journals there exist opposing studies by prestigious institutes denying the connection between UV light and cataracts, pterygiums and skin cancer. On the other hand, evidence exists that humans need some UV light both on the skin to produce vitamin D and through the eyes to regulate health and happiness. Putting infants and children into sunglasses to prevent senile cataracts and pterygiums may actually have harmful side effects now.

Light food for thought

Sunlight is a natural antibiotic; it destroys certain bacteria, fungi and viruses. It prevents and heals jaundice, the inability of immature livers to detoxify bilirubin, a yellow pigment produced by dying red blood cells. The sensible thing to do with babies with jaundice would be to put them in sunlight for short periods. Babies born in hospitals spend their first few days in windowless nurseries. Those who develop jaundice are blindfolded and placed under blue fluorescent lights, a costly procedure. Giving newborns a bit of sunlight was the original cure for jaundice, and could also prevent it.

Humans are diurnal creatures. Humans are awake during the day and asleep at night, unlike the more nocturnal kangaroos and echidnas that party around my garden at night. This means that people's mental, emotional and physical rhythms are attuned to daily sunlight.

UV light, or lack of it, affects hormone cycles. Nurses who work night shifts and sleep during the day find their periods become abnormal and irregular. Children who attend school in buildings without windows, under fluorescent lights, show more sexual aberrations than those in rooms with windows. In Germany an architect designed a home without windows for the blind. The structure had to be promptly rebuilt. The inhabitants were getting ill from light starvation.

Sunlight on skin is necessary for vitamin D production. By 1900 the industrial cities of the world were covered by a thick blanket of smoke. Ninety percent of the children in those cities suffered from rickets; their bones were soft and deformed. Make sure your children get some sunlight on their bodies — and please don't *over*-soap them. Natural vitamin D is formed by the interaction of UV light with oils produced on the skin's surface. Washing with soap removes this oil. Is that why some children hate to wash? The artificial vitamin D added to milk does not have the same chemical structure as the vitamin D made by skin and UV light.

Stimulation of the endocrine system (pineal, pituitary, thyroid, parathyroid, pancreas, spleen, adrenals and gonads) which rules growth in children, sexual behaviour, appetite, mood, temperature, and metabolism occurs through the retina of the eye. Therefore some optometrists recommend glasses that **do not** block UV light into the eyes.

Zane Kime MD, author of 'Sunlight Can Save Your Life', feels that UV light in the proper amount is **essential for prevention of skin cancer.** Wearing sunglasses may prevent your skin from getting the message to produce protective *melanin* — a prevention to skin cancer. Kime recommends gradual and moderate tanning of the skin. The only agreement is that no one should ever sunburn their skin or their eyes. Cancer cells love to multiply in an anaerobic environment. Scar tissue from long-past sunburns provides such a low oxygen medium.

You can make sure your children do not get sunburned, by covering them with clothing when they are outdoors. Kime recommends **not** using sunblocks. Slathering oils and preservatives on the skin smothers breathing pores and lends a false illusion of safety on the beach. A new sunblock has entered the market and is described as 'non-chemical'. Titanium dioxide flecks in this product reflect the UV light like tiny mirrors. It sounds superior to chemical UV absorbers. However, after short and sensible exposure of skin, it may be far better to cover up with clothing, wear a hat and find the trees.

The National Council for Prevention of Cancer in the US recommends that people do not use sunglasses or sunblock. An odd possibility rears its amazing head. Could it be possible that the current medical and government policy of recommending sunblocks and wearing sunglasses may itself be contributing to the incidence of skin cancer?

Why eyes need sunlight

Retinal nerve cells respond only to light. Light is their food. Fish in caves and burros in mines become blind from lack of light. You certainly won't go blind from using sunglasses but have you noticed loss of light tolerance? In 1967 I travelled to the Caribbean sporting prescription sunglasses. In the night a native sat on my backpack, smashing my glasses. The next morning I was stunned and incapacitated by the glare off sand and water. Since that time I have never worn sunglasses, not even to drive into the setting sun on Los Angeles freeways surrounded by 12 lanes of shiny clean cars. I sun my eyes in small doses at every opportunity. If you do Sunning each day for two weeks you may no longer be bothered by glare, nor will you be squinting in the light.

After Sunning vision is clearer and details are brighter. Kindly realise that Sunning does not mean staring with open eyes directly into the sun, as many eye professionals falsely assume. Sunning consists of closing your eyes and with relaxation moving your head around, circling the sun for ten minutes or less. You take in no more UV light than you would walking down the street or hanging clothes on the line.

The benefit is tremendous. A daily dose of UV light is supplied. The sun's warmth relaxes tight eye muscles. Retinal cells are stimulated; glare is reduced and dispositions turn - sunny.

Sunning games

Sit or stand comfortably facing the sun. Morning or afternoon is best; not high noon when the sun is directly overhead. If the sun is too bright, do your Sunning in a shady area.

Close your eyes and pretend the sun is a huge sunflower. Put a Magic Nose Feather on the end of your nose. With your Magic Feather make a circle on top of the sunflower petals. Rotate your

Help Your Child to Perfect Eyesight

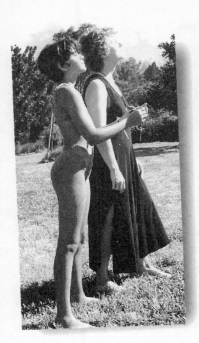

Alexandra and NVI teacher Isabele Steiner (Switz.) sunning

whole head slowly, gently. Whisper 'thank you' to the sun for its free gift of warmth and light and life upon the earth. Occasionally change the colour of your Magic Nose Feather and sunflower to sunkissed orange; to cherry red; to sapphire blue.

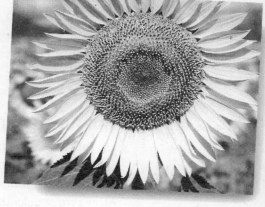

A sunflower

Make a Sun Sandwich

After Sunning for a minute, Palm your eyes (page 123) and watch the brilliant light show that appears as after-images dissolve from orange to red to magenta. When the light show finally slows to deep black, Sun again for a minute. Repeat the Palming. Colours will become more dramatic and

Sunning Song

Words and Music by Bernard O'Scanaill

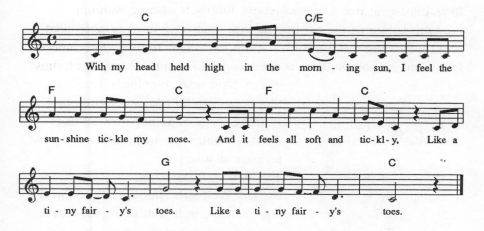

With my head held high in the morn - ing sun, I feel the sun-shine tic-kle my nose. And it feels all soft and tic-kl-y, Like a ti - ny fair - y's toes. Like a ti - ny fair - y's toes.

With my head held high in the morning sun,
I feel the sunshine tickle my chin.
And it makes me feel all smily,
Like a tiny fairy grin.
Like a tiny fairy grin.

your black will go velvety, like a black panther.

Make a Suncup

Hold your palms cupped, facing the sun so that you feel its heat and light in the centre of your hands. After your hands are filled with sunlight, pour the light into your eyes. Let your eyes have a long drink of light out of your hands. End with Palming.

Colour therapy

In the psycho-pharmacology department, University of Melbourne, Trevor Norman sets depressed people under strong white light for two hours each day. Every minute they glance at the light. After two weeks their SADness (Seasonal Affective Disorder) is relieved. He believes that the blue-green wave length entering eyes regulates levels of the hormone *melatonin*. Melatonin levels increase in the evening when the sun goes down and decrease at sunrise. Daily Sunning for five minutes could have the same uplifting effect. Natural sunlight contains all colour wavelengths. You will be taking in the blue-green wave while Sunning.

Blue Lagoon

To set up a blue-green experience with your children, use theatre gels or coloured transparency paper from a stationery shop placed in front of an ordinary incandescent light bulb. Or hold coloured paper in front of your faces while Sunning. Imagine you are in a lagoon, swimming with fishes and mermaids. You could be at the Great Barrier Reef, exploring wrecked rusty ships, finding sunken treasure.

Each colour of the rainbow affects your feelings. A bright yellow room will wake you up. A blue room, especially in turquoise shades, will calm and soothe. Blue is the accepted healing colour for eyes and

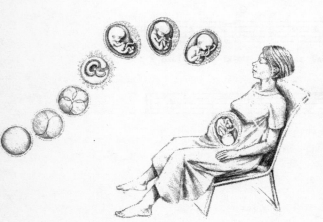

vision. Blue skies, bluebirds, bluebells, blue frogs can be imagined while Palming (page 123). See how colour from the sun, your imagination and your feelings all interplay.

Pre-birth Sunning

In 'The Well Baby Book', Mike Samuels MD recommends that expecting mamas expose their belly to direct sunlight. The effect on the baby in utero is stimulation of visual perception. At seven months all senses are receiving.

👁 Help Your Child to Perfect Eyesight

Your yet to be born child hears you humming and singing, while absorbing the vibrations of light.

Scared of the dark

Many children (and adults too) are afraid of the dark. When eight year-old Jack switched off his brain while looking at a black crayon, his whole family engaged in drawing and story telling to resolve the issue. Jack's younger sisters had to escort him to the outdoor toilet at night. This came out as we all sat on the floor sketching with crayons on large sheets of paper. The instructions were to draw a night-time picture on one half of the sheet and a daytime view on the other half.

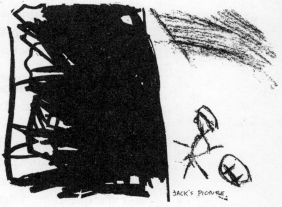

Jack's drawing of night and day

Jack's night side is completely covered with crayon: no images, only jet black obscurity. His daytime drawing shows blue sky, himself, a football. By contrast his four year-old sister's night drawing shows her house, stars and a crescent moon. The sunny day side is drawn completely in yellow crayon, with a boat riding on yellow waves. What is fascinating is her name: the first letters E and m are drawn in black; the following m and a are in daylight yellow. She is at peace with the duality of day and night within herself.

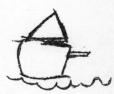

Emma's drawing of night and day

I suggest doing the drawing game of day and night with all children. If any fears are expressed verbally or with black crayon, do the Melting Beachballs games. For a full explanation of this procedure, skip forward to page 136.

Positive	Negative
I love the light	I'm afraid of the light
I love the darkness	I'm afraid of the dark

Place the phrase 'I love the light' in your left hand. Imagine a large yellow beach ball in your palm. Repeat the words, 'I love the light.' Allow your memories about the sun coming up in the morning and illuminating the world to flow freely. Intensify all the feelings, either those that say, 'The flowers are growing because of the light' or 'Actually I hate to get up in the morning and go to school, and do my chores and suffer.' When you have explored your feelings about light to your satisfaction and blown your yellow beach ball up to world class proportions, put the opposite in your right hand: 'I'm afraid of the light'. 'The cancer lady who came to school told us it makes holes in your skin. I will go blind if I go outdoors. You must never go outdoors in the sun.' (These statements came from a five year-old after her school was visited by a well-intentioned Anti-Cancer Society lecturer.)

Once all social input and inner fears have been voiced and magnified (celebrated), then you ask the questions, 'Is it OK to be afraid of the light?' and 'Is it OK to love the light?'. When the answer on both sides is 'Yes', bring your two beach balls together at your heart. Do the same process using the sentences, 'I love the darkness' and 'I'm afraid of the dark.' When magnifying the beachball you can ask the question, 'What happens in the light?' or 'What happens in the darkness?' to coax out any shy thought-gnomes that may feel it's not safe to show themselves. After doing Melting Beachballs with light and dark, see if behaviour alters in relationship to necessary, solitary trips into darkness. See if irrational fears about either sunlight or darkness, both of which relate to life and death themes, are softened or dissolved.

Timetable for sunning

birth to two years +

Babies and toddlers need ten minutes of sunlight on their skin for vitamin D production and pituitary stimulation. After that they must be completely protected by clothing and a sunhat from any degree of sunburn.

two to six years

Two year-olds will imitate anything, including people closing their eyes and making circles around the sun. When they are ready voice a 'Thank you' to the sun for its life-giving force. Introduce painting colours with total 'hands on' enthusiasm.

six to 12+ years

Circle on imaginary sunflowers with closed eyes. Invent new Sunning images together. Create a balanced rational attitude toward UV light; neither too much exposure nor too little: neither irrational fear nor disrespect for its power.

Help Your Child to Perfect Eyesight

Chapter Ten

Children relax with imagination and colour

Are children relaxed?

Inside children with visual blur there is a room where they are tied up in knots. This room could be well hidden. Little myopes perform well in school. They laugh, make jokes, engage in sports. A hyperopic child with eye coordination problems catches up with her class when she puts on magnifying lenses. It looks as if we have a happy, well-adjusted child once she gets the correct glasses. But there's still that hidden room.

It is my hope that with the help of this book you and your child will be able to find that hidden room; open doors, unlock drawers and sweep away stress. This is of greater value to me than knowing that your child is performing to social standards.

This chapter gives you more ideas for relaxation games that can be linked to home and school activities. Everyone's creativity, communication and joy in living will go up a notch as well as their visual acuity. Relaxing and imagining gives everyone courage and strength for opening closed rooms.

Relaxation comes from activating the right hemisphere of the brain. Relaxation does not mean collapsing and falling asleep. True relaxation is a state of dynamic softness and receptivity. Relaxed minds are natural springs of bright ideas and bubbling wit; unrestrained by competition and correction. Relaxed eyes light up. Life energy freely circulates through the whole visual system.

Engaging in a free-flow of pleasant images produces relaxation. Everyone has these imaging abilities built in. It is not necessary to take a drug to visualize. The river of images will have a theme and a direction. The images are never wrong. If someone puts purple spots on an eagle and sets him down to drink dirty sock tea with a whale in the middle of the oven, then that's the way it is. Brain-storming sessions in high-tech corporations have three rules. Firstly, all ideas are correct; there are no scornful voices saying, 'That's unrealistic.' Secondly, wild and zany ideas are encouraged. Thirdly, the more ideas the better. During a NVI teachers' conference, we brain-stormed ways to do the Bird of a Feather Swing with trees. The list reached 124 possibilities. It was difficult to stop and go home.

Please do not allow anyone to mess with imagery games using a left-brain compulsion to correct and be rational. A friend in Los Angeles asked his four year-old where kangaroo mothers carry their babies. She replied, 'in their mouth.' Dad chided, 'No, you know better than that. Kangaroos carry their babies in their pouch.' Tracey had never seen a kangaroo. Her dad had never seen our local endangered frog that carries its babies in its mouth.

If your child is already caught up in the habit of worrying, if she projects negative futures, the following games will be most helpful. This child could use a story that addresses both her inner nervousness and helps her gain control of her imagination. All children need skills to accept and change the images parading through their minds. Children are open receivers. They witness adult soap operas at home and on the screen. They read books and talk to other children. By the age of six, youthful memory banks are crowded with video store categories; horror, comedy, romantic drama, action chases, science fiction, war documentaries. These films need to be coaxed out, reviewed, transmuted and defused if your child is being controlled or affected by them.

Home again in the self

A child who respects and uses her imagination becomes very independent. You as an adult may have to get used to going inside your own head in order to meet the child who is already in hers. Imagination has been schooled out of most adults. When did you stop drawing? At what age did you stop writing stories? You can regress back to that stage and start up again with painting pictures in your mind. Never mind if your paints are all dried up.

If parents are too busy to laze around with their child or to take 15 minutes for a heart-to-heart talk, children will seek stimulation or anaesthesia elsewhere. Television sets have become baby-sitters and pseudo entertainers. The amount of time children spend watching television means they are not spending time with their own life process.

Television becomes a substitute for personal imagination and sharing inner worlds. If a child has an active inner life which is shared with the world at large, watching TV will be too boring. Replace some of your child's TV watching time with your time. Let the housework or golf game go.

Imagining with Palming

Palming is an ancient technique for healing eyes. I can see the Flintstones lying around a firepit, Palming and telling dinosaur stories. Yogis have been Palming their eyes for several thousand years. I don't know what pictures they had going through their minds!

Palming sends healing energy from warm hands into eyes and mind. When Palming you have nowhere else to go except inside yourself. Shutting off all outside light stimulation rests retinal cells and gives you a break from the obligations of the outside world.

Most people think that imagining does not affect the visual system. The latest in scientific research confirms the opposite is true. When you imagine a horse running across the plains, your foot kicking a ball or the smell of a red rose, electricity and blood circulation increase in your visual brain. Generating internal images causes bodily changes. This fact is used constantly in Natural Vision Improvement to relax muscles, to establish fusion and generally restore brilliant clear eyesight.

How to Palm

Cup your hands and place them over your eyes so that all outside light is shut out. I like to close my eyes under my palms. Then you do your best to turn off thinking and turn on your inner movies. You can do this alone or you can make a Palming Circle with friends.

Palming variations

- Someone read a book while others are Palming.
- Someone start a story and pass it to the next person.
- Someone choose a colour; everything imagined has to be in that colour.
- Someone choose a theme such as animals or sports; everyone has to tell about an animal or game they are seeing in their own mind.
- Smells will bring out memory pictures in your mind faster than anything else. One person gather some smelly things together and hold them under the nose of the person who is Palming. Suggestions: fresh grass, a flower, vanilla essence or some cooking oil on tissue paper, some

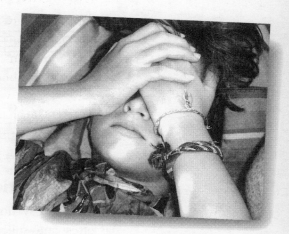

What is Claire imagining?

cinnamon or soap. Ask the question, 'What does this smell remind you of?'

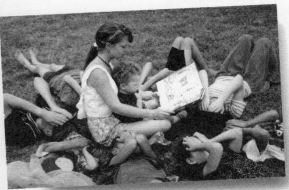

Carina reads a story for her Palming Circle

• Combine Sketching with Palming. As images rise up behind your closed eyes, sketch them with your Magic Nose Pencil. This will bring together movement and relaxation.

• Draw a big house inside your mind, containing lots of different kinds of food for different sorts of animals. What kind of food do you have in your house? Hay? What sort of animal would like to come in the door and eat that hay? What sound does this animal make? Take turns with this game.

When I'm Palming

Words and Melody by Janet Goodrich

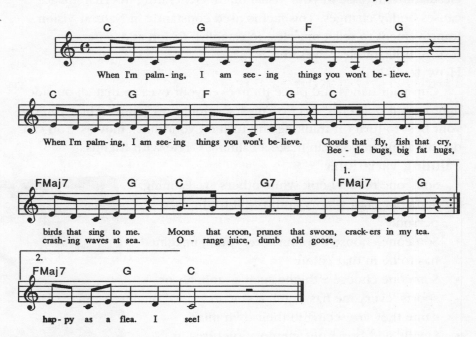

When I'm palm-ing, I am see-ing things you won't be-lieve.

When I'm palm-ing, I am see-ing things you won't be-lieve. Clouds that fly, fish that cry, / Bee - tle bugs, big fat hugs,

birds that sing to me. Moons that croon, prunes that swoon, crack-ers in my tea. / crash-ing waves at sea. O - range juice, dumb old goose,

hap-py as a flea. I see!

Auto-suggestion training

Used by psychologists, psychiatrists and producers of meditation cassettes, auto-suggestion consists of repeated verbal phrases that deliberately release muscles and deepen breathing. The autonomic nervous system responds instantly to auto-suggestion. Cold hands and

👁 Help Your Child to Perfect Eyesight

feet turn warm; a mild tingling sensation is felt; contracted muscles lengthen. Child therapist and counsellor Else Mueller has written books to read to children at bedtime. Her stories are framed by auto-suggestions and the characters within the story are taken through a process of relaxation - including the elves and frogs. I would add Palming to the process.

Bedtime story

Everyone lie down except for the person who is reading slowly and soothingly. Use the following suggestions before each bedtime story. Your child's arms may come down and hands fall away from her face. That's OK. Sleep comes quickly. If you tell a story during the day when melatonin levels are close to zero, an older child will relax deeply while her mind stays alert.

'Your legs are growing very long. Your back is relaxed and long. Feel how heavy your body is. Your arms are getting long. Your arms are lighter than air. They float upward and bend at the elbows, so your hands fall gently over your closed eyes. All the light is closed out. It's like going into a warm, soft cave where everything is dark. Here comes a story.

The Ugly Duckling Story

Mother Duck proudly looked over the five white eggs in her nest beside the pond. Every day she spread her warm brown feathers over them and closed her eyes, dreaming of the cute little yellow ducklings that would soon follow her down to the water to swim. One morning after nibbling on grass blades and swallowing a black beetle, Mother Duck returned to her nest to dream again of her new family. She did not notice the sixth egg that was nestled amongst the others. Ducks can only count up to five.

On a dewy spring morning, Mother Duck woke up and lifted one orange foot high in the air. She had heard a cracking sound. The first duckling was pecking his way through the eggshell. Mother duck waddled off her nest. With happy eyes she watched bits of eggshell flying in all directions. Her babies were hatching. She clucked and clicked and chuckled. She wanted her ducklings to hear her voice first so they would always come when she called. Mother Duck wriggled her white tail feathers over their heads so they would learn the shape of her rear end and always follow her when she moved. The soft morning sun dried the ducklings' wet downy feathers. Each duckling turned into a cute yellow ball of fluff with precious little orange legs and alert, beady eyes.

All except the sixth duckling. When she was sun dried her feathers were dull grey. Her legs were long and clumsy. Her eyes rolled around in all directions. Mother Duck turned her head from side to side as she scanned this duckling. She wondered if this one really belonged in her family. Deciding that a duckling is a duckling no matter what colour or what size it is, Mother Duck waddled down to the water's edge. Five cute ducklings and one ugly duckling followed her white tail feathers and her quacking voice right into the water for their first swim.

The next day other animals and the farmer's children came round to see the freshly hatched ducklings. They OOH-ed and AAH-ed over the five cute fluffy ducklings with their little orange feet. They frowned and threw stones and sticks at the grey, googly-eyed duckling.

The Ugly Duckling let her head droop. She wandered away from the nest, shedding big hot tears from her sad eyes. 'Nobody loves me,' she said to the empty blue sky. 'Nobody wants me,' she moaned in the cool black night. 'I'm terribly ugly,' she screamed at the silent hard sun.

The Ugly Duckling wandered alone over hills, down roads, through cities, across fields. Everywhere people said, 'Scat!' Animals said, 'Shoo!' The trees and flowers said nothing.

Winter came, snow flakes fell from the sky. The Ugly Duckling shivered by a pond covered with a thick

Help Your Child to Perfect Eyesight

layer of ice. She let her wings droop. Her shoulders softened. She closed her eyes. She imagined warm summer sun stroking her feathers. Feel how heavy her body became. She sank into the ground. At the same time she grew bigger until she filled the whole sky. Her breathing became very slow; feel her long deep breaths.

She looked upward into softly falling snow. One snowflake grew wings - great white wings that flapped and made a wind on her face. The huge bird that owned these snow-white wings landed right next to her. The Ugly Duckling was afraid to speak to such a beautiful large bird. 'Hello,' said the graceful long-necked swan. 'I saw you down here by yourself. Can't imagine why you'd be alone at a time like this. Just when the coldest weather is coming. Where's your nest? Where's your family? What's your name? What kind of fish swim in this pond? What's the matter? Cat got your tongue?' The Ugly Duckling could only say, 'AUGHH.' Her voice was rusty from not being used. 'AUGHH,' she croaked. 'Me. Ugly. Duckling. Googly-eyes.'

The beautiful swan flapped her wings, turned around three times in the mud on her strong black legs and laughed. 'You, ugly? That's funny. What a joke. Here tickle me again right under my wing. HO HA. You are one of the more handsome of us, I would say. Go have a look in the pond.'

The Ugly Duckling peeked shyly into the glassy surface of the water. She turned her head from side to side. She saw a long white neck, two straight eyes and strong white wings. 'Am I you?' She asked the swan. 'Am I big and gorgeous like you?' 'Yes, yes, yes,' said the big friendly swan. 'Come along now and meet the others. You can join our nest and cuddle up with the rest of us. It's going to be a chilly black night.'

Colour all your life

Imagining with Palming improves eyesight. Imagining colours while Palming will make Cone Phones ring. Colour is made in our minds. There is no colour in the outside world, just light beams from the sun or artificial lights bouncing around in space. The same cone phones that register colour wavelengths also tell the visual brain about sharp details. If you are able to imagine colour in your mind, you will perceive colour and details more easily when your eyes are open.

With your eyes closed, make a noise and ask yourself and everyone else what colour the noise is. See that colour in your mind. Repeat the process. Listen to music and make the music into colours.

Emotional healing for imagining

Is being imaginative safe? One powerful reason why children cut off their imagination is out of fear. A good many of these fears can be traced to the method of education or picked up from parents. For example:

If I imagine too much...

no one will like me.

I will go crazy and be taken away to the looney bin.

I will be different from everyone else, I won't fit in.

I will not give the answers the teachers want.

my Dad won't love me.

As a family, explore everyone's fears about being wildly imaginative. In the business world creative imaging and wild fantasising is called 'lateral thinking'. People who dare to do it are well paid. Use Melting Beachballs on page 136 to tame your fear of unbridled imagination.

Scary stories

Saying 'no' to your child when she wants to watch horror movies is your prerogative. But please do not ignore the fact that she probably already has a few in her head. The following imagery games may be useful in this case. Some children remain eternally silent about what scares them the most. Frightening images control children if they are not brought out in the open. Nightmare-causing memories can be disarmed with the following activities:

What happens next?

Everyone lies down and Palms. The leader asks this question: 'What is the scariest thing you can think of?'

When everyone has responded, the leader asks, 'What's the worst thing that can happen?'

When replies are flowing, keep the questions going: 'Yes, and what happens next? ...and after that what happens?'

Often this spontaneous and uncensored movie-making will reveal surprising, maybe shocking images. Be careful not to judge. Today's children are plugged into a culture that does not monitor their minds for damage. It's up to you to give them the tools, even if you think they are 'too young' to be dealing with certain images. If monsters arise, play the Sculpting Monsters game. Two can play, three or more will add to the action.

Sculpting Monsters

Continue Palming and drawing all the images that come into your mind with your Magic Nose Pencils. Start a co-operative monster creation. One person might begin with, 'I see a leg. This leg is like a tree trunk, only it is orange and covered with hairs and warts. It is stomping around by itself, moaning, "Where is my arm?"' The next person adds an arm to the monster, a horrible arm. A third person could contribute a head or heads. After the monster is sculpted, the important decision has to be reached: **What do we do with the monster?** Brain-storm this question.

Do we sprinkle holy water over it so it melts away? Do we make friends with it and ask it to dinner? Shall we enter into and become the monster, to experience what it's like in there? (It could be sad and lonely.) What about chopping it to pieces and eating it with strawberry sauce?

You may give your child some suggestions to make it OK to resolve monsters but the final solution must be hers. Ask her if she is satisfied at the end. If she isn't, have her spend some time with this question and give you the answer later. It may come in her dreams. Children who have nightmares can benefit greatly by being given a few

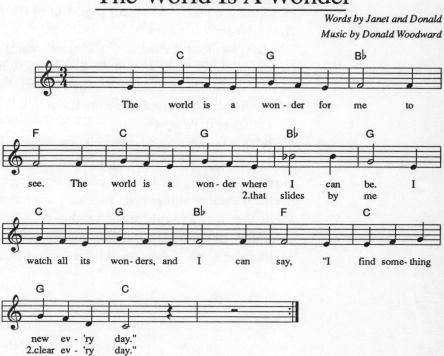

The World Is A Wonder

Words by Janet and Donald
Music by Donald Woodward

The world is a won-der for me to see. The world is a won-der where I can be. I
2.that slides by me
watch all its won-ders, and I can say, "I find some-thing
new ev-'ry day."
2.clear ev-'ry day."

conscious tools to use in their dream state. When confronted by scary images, they can take control in their dream by turning to the monster and saying, 'What are you doing here and what do you want?'

Sing The World is a Wonder (on previous page) to restore a sense of appreciation about everything you see.

Timetable for colours and imagining

birth to one year +

When given a choice, most young children will choose red. If you are playing vision games with a purpose, such as Favouring the Phoria in strabismus (page 189), make a collection of red objects: a cloth ball, a red plastic spoon, a red scarf, a red feather. Use these red objects in your directional games with the child. Red is not a requirement, your child may go for yellow or blue.

one to three years +

Let the child pick out her own clothes and toys. Red again? Place red objects around the room and drape a red scarf over a picture frame. Put a red button on the table top. Show your child one red object, then have her close her eyes and imagine red. Ask her to go find all the red objects you've placed in the room. With an older child, have her paint the room with her red Nose Paint Brush, exclaiming when a red object pops out of the background.

three to seven years+

Have a colour theme day. 'Today let's paint only with blue'. Finger paints are super. Have lots of paper and see what happens. Read picture books aloud. Feel free to describe the images on the page while your child Palms and paints them in her mind.

seven to ten years+

What's your favourite colour? Let's make vision game tools in this colour: a magic wand with a purple ribbon. An eyepatch decorated in purple. A drawing book full of purple drawings. A dress-up day in purple. Palming with purple, picking purple flowers. Use a purple Magic Pencil or a purple Magic Feather on purple noses. Palming continues. Emotional Healing for imagination may be advisable as most adults remember they stopped drawing and visualising at this age.

Chapter Eleven

Feelings and eyesight

What do you feel?

'I don't want a lot of people to know about when I wore glasses. It was horrible. I was never really together with my friends when they played games. I always had to think about where to put my glasses.

'I was frightened about them breaking and of glass going in my eye. That's funny. I am frightened about my left eye. It doesn't feel part of me. When the vision teacher did some work to use both eyes together I was frightened. Maybe I wouldn't be able to see. I don't know what seeing means. It would be very nice to see.

'I wasn't very good at sport. I didn't know why. I tried very hard but sometimes I made a mistake, like in catching a ball. I just couldn't do it and it made me very unhappy. I don't remember the operation. I don't really like all those people for giving me glasses I didn't need. I was always called names too. I don't like being called names.' — Eric Kiernan, Aikido teacher, speaking from his inner child.

Why do the vast majority of people who put children into glasses ignore the inner child? Perhaps their own childhood is bottled and sealed. Every child is chock full, of feelings. Vacuum packed, childhood feelings are preserved into adulthood. Different years have different vintages. Let us devise a small game that may help every child keep his inner self ever fresh - without the canning process.

Body posture, facial expressions, free or stiff movements of limbs and especially the look in the eyes, comprise a graphic non-verbal communication which comes before proper spoken language. Is this child sad, happy, irritated, bored, vivacious, angry, or scared? His eyes will tell you if his expression is not completely locked and deadened behind glasses.

Seven emotions

For me the emotional health of children has more value than social correctness. The result is happy resilient adults who relate to one another in conscious empathy.

Joy and love, pain, anger, fear, sadness, apathy and unconsciousness each have an energy vibration and a core statement which can be voiced. Everyone cycles continually through all seven emotions. When you linger too long in a vibratory feeling and thinking pattern other than joy, you develop what is called an 'emotional problem'.

There are many shades of emotions, all variations on the major seven. Everyone's primal state is joy. Creation brings us into life on a wave of joy and love. A return to health and happiness necessitates a return journey through whatever feelings were judged and suppressed in childhood. Seeing clearly without glasses is unrestricted enjoyment of your visual system. It is normal for vision to falter occasionally. It is normal for vision to bounce back readily in the same way a small child is sad one moment and sunny the next.

Joy

...verbally expresses itself as 'I love that'; 'Isn't that beautiful?'; 'That's wonderful.' Joy is the state of being in love with everything all the time. Our whole system was designed to continually return to this level after flowing through the other human feelings. If joy is judged and dampened then you may feel...

Pain

You are in pain if you feel less than a calm joyful appreciation about anything. Your pain can be physical, emotional, mental or spiritual.

Pain expresses itself verbally as 'It hurts.' The child is blessed whose parents teach him how to accept and transmute pain, rather than anaesthetise or reject it physically and mentally. 'Don't cry.' 'It doesn't hurt.' 'Just get over it.' Experiment with the message, 'Love your pain. What is it showing you?' Children are naturally adept at transmuting pain back to joy unless they learn that pain is bad and must be buried.

If pain is judged as bad (and children pick up attitudes toward pain by the time they are one year old), then the pain level is submerged and you may experience...

Anger

Yes, children do get angry. Repressed anger can re-emerge as hyperopia and crossed eyes. These are children who can throw champion temper tantrums. When doing vision games with these children, kindly make the room and your psyche reaction-proof. Make sure everything the child might touch is hardy. Have lots of pillows and cushions for pouncing and pounding when the urge to take action appears. 'My, what a wonderful roaring lion you are!' Set limits in the midst of chaos. The first limit is the sanctity of someone else's body. 'Don't hit your little sister, hit the couch.' The trust that the child's life energy will bring him back to a state of tranquillity will allow you to put up with free expression of anger.

When anger is suppressed it comes out mentally as '**I'm right** about this and **you are wrong**.' Some phrases heard when suppressed anger rules the personality are: 'The doctors are right and everyone else, including you and your intuitive feelings, is wrong' or 'There is no scientific proof and your own experience is not proof enough' or 'Those blankedy-blank doctors ruined my (her, his, their) eyes.' Don't blame the doctors. Be angry, express it and rise to pain and joy. Your power to act and influence reality returns.

If anger is not permitted at all then the vibrations of the child may slow down to...

Fear

Fear says or thinks, 'I'm scared I will do it wrong' or 'Are you sure you're doing the right thing?' or 'What if we only do vision games and our child goes blind?' Myopes are constantly struggling with the fear of not being perfect in society, in school or with friends. Myopes become masters at hiding their fear, eventually even from themselves.

If fear is not accepted and befriended, then your whole mind and body will sink into...

Sadness

Sadness makes children tired if tears are not completely shed with great enthusiasm. Chronic fatigue syndrome can appear later in adolescence and adulthood. It is better to encourage full crying now, until sunbeams re-emerge from behind sad, heavy clouds. Expressions of sadness find their way into left-brain time-linked utterances such as 'I'll **always** be like this'or 'He will **never** see clearly.'

If boys and girls don't cry then the human organism may experience...

Apathy

Apathy expresses itself in thoughts or utterances such as, 'You can't do that.' 'I'm sorry, Mrs. Smith, there is nothing that can be done about your child's eyes.' 'Science knows that nothing works' or 'It doesn't matter.' The nicest people are apathetic in their confident assurance that you just cannot change this child's vision.

If we judge and hate the apathy in others or ourselves, then we get so wiped out we fall right into...

Unconsciousness

Here is the repository of all our forgotten wisdom, remedies, healing techniques. **'I don't know** what to do.' or 'My grandmother had some answer for this, but **I've forgotten** what she did.' Here we don't feel pain any longer, nor perceive much. It's a safe place to hang out but it does result in a robotic society. All anaesthesias put us at this level, including the ones sold over the counters.

Unconsciousness: the walking dead, Zombiville. Most of us live here. This is the worship of technological response. Cut it out. Cover it. Drug it. Make it stop. Go to sleep. Forget about it. Deny it. It doesn't exist. It has no validity. It isn't scientific.

The only way out of the valley of unconsciousness that prevails in our 'it's normal to be sick' society is to be in a state of wonder about it. Everything that exists is a miracle, no matter how awful it may appear. Then our life energy jumps right back up to joy.

A child comes into life with heaps of flexibility. He cries and then smiles, he sleeps and is ready to go again; he uses emotion as a playground. Suspend the judge.

Eyes talk

Eyes communicate with one another continually. This silent language can be more powerful than words. Deadness of expression in the eyes means outgoing messages has been stifled and feelings are no longer being expressed directly. When people first take off their glasses they are not only afraid of making mistakes, they are also frightened of allowing a tear or a spark of anger to show. Take away the fear and the eyes begin to talk once more. What do they say?

Psychologists have observed the way bosses and underlings use their eyes. A manager's extended stare communicates, 'I'm stronger and bigger than you.' Workers avert their eyes, admitting, 'I'm guilty' or 'I'm intimidated.' Playing a dominant role requires hiding emotions while the subordinate player must display his nervousness and tense his shoulders and drop his head.

This scenario is enacted in offices, classrooms and at home. If you are aware of the game being played through silent visual communications you have a behaviour choice. You can take it seriously at the risk of all the actors getting hypnotised by their roles; or you can remark on and mime the communication gestures. Playing with eye talk will free everyone to change their language. If you have a goal of treating others as equals, including children, then awareness of unconscious eye and body language will bring you closer to that aim. Notice how eyes talk in your family. You and your children's visual expression can be explored in all its subtleties and allowed to develop without fear or withdrawal. Good vision includes direct communication from eye to eye.

I Can Be...

Words by Janet Goodrich

Music by Donald Woodward

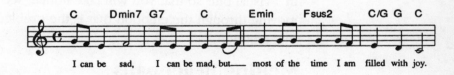

I can be sad, I can be mad, but most of the time I am filled with joy.

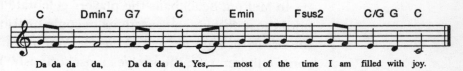

Da da da da, Da da da da, Yes, most of the time I am filled with joy.

I can be scared,
I can be brave,
but most of the time I am filled with joy.
Da, da, da, da,
Da ,da, da ,da,
Yes, most of the time I am filled with joy.

I can be blue,
I can be brown,
but most of the time I am filled with joy.
Da, da, da, da,
Da ,da, da ,da,
Yes, most of the time I am filled with joy.

Make up your own words!!

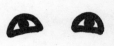
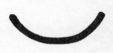

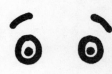

Everyone can develop more emotional flexibility and more time in the hall of joy by exploring candidly what comes up. To set the stage for this, you could play with recognizing and celebrating different emotional states.

Playacting

Each person does an emotion for three to four minutes then passes it on to another person who represents another emotion.

Teach children the common words and phrases they will hear with each brand of bottled up feeling.

anger	'He did it.'
sadness	'She always takes my crayon'
apathy	'I don't care'
unconsciousness	'I forgot. I don't remember'.

Read stories which express emotions while the children are Palming. They will be glad to contribute sound effects.

With the following emotional healing game it may be possible to help every child loosen up emotionally and stay loose. Children will seek help from you by being annoying, withdrawn, obnoxious, ill or in a visual blur so that you will take notice, see and help. It's not moving through the emotion that is the problem. It's getting stuck in that emotion.

Melting Beachballs

In Melting Beachballs the players celebrate negative feelings until those forbidden sensations become hilarious. This levity is the break-through we're looking for. You may have noticed that some children take themselves most seriously. This is where we want to uncover natural levity - a lightness of being inherent in every person. This is not teasing, ridiculing or denying but a true celebration of what is. Often what is there is self-hate. **If people disapprove that I hate myself, I will bury it even deeper with my little shovel.** Once we dig up hate and take a good look at this truly unpleasant feeling and state of mind, then we can ask, 'What is the opposite of hating myself?' Do not ask this latter question **too early** in the game or someone will think you have a preference.

You may think celebrating the negative gives it power. Please realise that self-negation is already there. Because it is also unacceptable it is hidden. This develops into a psychic canker in the smallest of children. Suppressed feelings control behaviour. Consider bringing out and celebrating the negative until it loses the power it has gained by being judged and closeted. Watch your child shine after his negatives have been released from the dungeon.

The following Emotional Healing game is based on **embracing the opposites in life.** Melting together hate and love, fear and courage, ugliness and beauty heals the split, the separation between our left and right halves, between mind and body. If you are even slightly successful with this game you will notice a lessening of tension in your child's body and in his eyes.

A child in its original state of Grace doesn't choose sides in any fight. Through these games children can learn to actually manipulate fear or anger and consciously bring in states of pleasure and joy. When taught this useful trick at a young age, you will find your teenagers priding themselves on how they can sit on a rock alone, resolving their own moods and problems.

👁 Help Your Child to Perfect Eyesight

The preliminary game: learning to melt opposites together — Angel and devil

I'm a little angel. I'm so good. Everybody loves me.

I'm a little devil. I'm naughty. I'm bad. Nobody loves me.

Put 'I'm a little angel' in your right hand in a big ball of energy. Put 'I'm a little devil' in your left hand in a big ball of energy. Switch back and forth, stating the message of each ball and making that ball bigger and stronger - until we sing, or whisper, or scream our message to the sky. When satisfied do-

The last move of the game

Squish and smoosh together slowly, passionately, your right hand ball and your left hand ball like Scarlett is doing in the photo below. Her physical beach balls won't blend together, but your imaginary ones will. They will come together like matter and anti-matter; perhaps with a BANG, a POOF, or a SHHHHH. Then interlace the fingers of your two hands together and bring them to the middle of your chest. Release your hands, your arms. Feel your lightness of being.

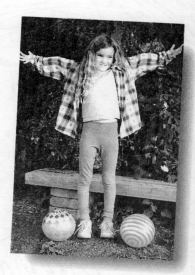

Scarlett is magnifying her Beachballs

Practise filling up and expanding beachballs with other opposites such as:

sad	happy
scared	brave
stupid	smart

SCARE·BRAVE   STUP·SMART

Become skilled at melting concepts together by practising with colours.

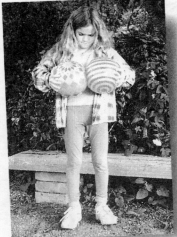

Scarlett smooshes her beachballs together

Choose a coloured crayon that feels like sad. With this colour make a big circle on a piece of paper. Colour in the circle so you have a beachball of solid blue, for example.

Hold the crayon in your hand and truly feel that colour. Close your eyes. Is it a heavy colour or a lightweight colour?

Now open your eyes and pick a crayon that feels like the opposite of sad. What does this colour feel like? Is it heavy or light weight? On a second sheet of paper make a solid beachball with this crayon.

Scarlett releases it all!

Hold your drawings in your hands, the sad colour in one hand and the happy colour in the other hand. Close your eyes. Imagine both balls growing huge - right off the paper.

Now bring your hands together, crumpling the paper. Imagine the colours are mixing together. What colour would this be?

Open your eyes and draw a beachball circle made of both colours on another paper. Put it on the wall and explain to your friends.

Take a deep breath

I have included breathing and yawning in this chapter about feeling and emotion because suppressed feelings are held in place by restricted breathing.

A child who freely breathes is a child whose emotions will flow quickly to a state of joy and openness.

Yawning frees the breath. Yawning releases tight jaws, tummies, and eyes. Yawning brightens and clears eyesight. Yawning increases oxygen supply to eyes and brain. Free breathers are clear seers.

Yawning with the Lions

Playact together:

A lion sits under a tree and yawns loud and lazily. He is

imagining what he would like
to eat. Off in the distance the lion sees something that might be
delicious, but he does not recognize exactly what it is. He wants
to stroll over there and find out if it would suit his tummy for
dinner. The lion stretches out his long front legs, then his long
back legs. He yawns again. Softly, carefully he crawls toward the
other creature; on all fours of course. Silently, feeling the ground
beneath his paws, he sneaks up on his dinner. Pouncing on his
dinner, the lion eats it all up with groans of pleasure and mighty
slurps. Yawn.

Huff-puff

A short, easy, breathing release for children who are already tied
up in knots and for all children to keep them emotionally free.

Duration: 30 seconds

When: during cuddle times or at bedtime

Position: with the child lying flat on his back on bed or floor or
on your lap

How: Place your hand lightly on your child's tummy. There
is a golden balloon inside this tummy. When your
child inhales the balloon gets bigger, the tummy fatter.
When he exhales, all the air in the balloon goes out.
We now have a flat tummy. Do this three times. With
small children that's enough. Adults have to breathe
for an hour to get the same effect.

Response: Ask him how he feels.

Tummy breathing slows down the heartbeat and stimulates a
right-brain, muscle-lengthening relaxation response.

Chest breathing stimulates a left-brain, hold-tight state in the body.

For good, balanced breathing and brain function we need both
tummy and chest movement.

Joyful seeing and singing

To the child

As you are growing and exploring with your eyes, ears, mouth
and fingers, the people who are caring for you play silly, silly
games with you. They hang bright, shiny things above you that
move in the wind. They put pictures up for you to play with, first
only with your eyes, then with your fingertips. They cuddle you
and sing to you. Later, you will sing these songs to yourself and
with your friends. You are a vision person.

The Goodness Song

Words and melody by Janet Goodrich
Music by Donald Woodward

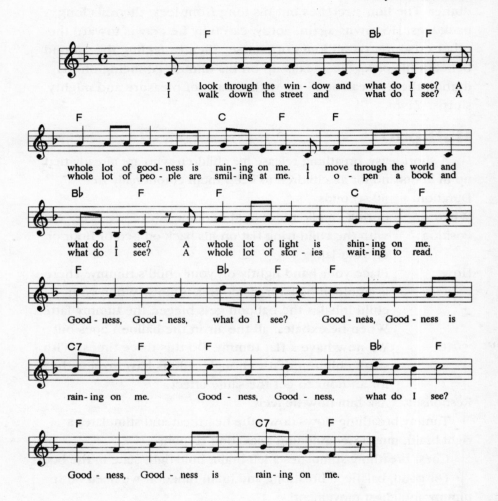

I look through the win - dow and what do I see? A
I walk down the street and what do I see? A

whole lot of good - ness is rain - ing on me. I move through the world and
whole lot of peo - ple are smil - ing at me. I o - pen a book and

what do I see? A whole lot of light is shin - ing on me.
what do I see? A whole lot of stor - ies wait - ing to read.

Good - ness, Good - ness, what do I see? Good - ness, Good - ness is

rain - ing on me. Good - ness, Good - ness, what do I see?

Good - ness, Good - ness is rain - ing on me.

Tell Me What You See

Lyrics by Janet Goodrich
Music based on a Prelude by Chopin

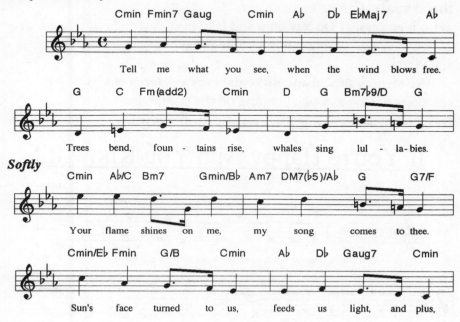

Slowly and Loudly

Cmin Fmin7 Gaug | Cmin Ab Db EbMaj7 | Ab

Tell me what you see, when the wind blows free.

G C Fm(add2) | Cmin D G Bm7b9/D | G

Trees bend, foun - tains rise, whales sing lul - la- bies.

Softly

Cmin Ab/C Bm7 | Gmin/Bb Am7 DM7(b5)/Ab | G G7/F

Your flame shines on me, my song comes to thee.

Cmin/Eb Fmin G/B | Cmin Ab Db Gaug7 | Cmin

Sun's face turned to us, feeds us light, and plus,

Still Softer

Cmin Ab/C Bmin7 | Gmin/Bb Am7 Ab7(b5 b9) G | G7/F

My child, I am yours, when all time and doors

Very Slowly

Cmin/Eb Fmin G/B | Cmin Ab Db Gaug7 | Cmin Cmin

O - pen wild - ly, God says, "We Shall See."

Timetable for emotional expression

birth to one year

Infants have feelings. Our society and upbringing calls for us to not know what to do for ourselves and to not express our feelings. Learn to receive the baby's cries of anger, fear and distress the best you can with supportive tranquillity even though I know you may be tired and grumpy yourself. Singing, toning, crooning, making noises with the child helps immensely. It carries your own tension away. If your jaw is tightening up and you're looking for an escape route, make noises with the kids. Hold the points from Chapter Six on yourself and your baby. Discover how soothing and freeing it can be. Apply love, forgiveness of self and others. Include the doctors.

three years +

Act out emotions: Do Yawning and Huff-puff,

Sing vision people songs.

six years +

Use Melting Beachballs, make the eyes and faces of seven emotions to look at while jumping on the trampoline.

Here is another song for joyful vision people

If You're Happy And You Know It

Traditional

If you're hap - py and you know it clap your hands; If you're

hap - py and you know it clap your hands; If you're

hap - py and you know it, then you real - ly ought to show it, If you're

hap - py and you know it clap your hands.

If you're happy and you know it do cross crawl...
If you're happy and you know it swing your head...
If you're happy and you know it blink a lot...
If you're happy and you know it sun your eyes...
If you're happy and you know it yawn out loud...
If you're happy and you know it palm your eyes...
If you're happy and you know it smile a lot...

Chapter Twelve

Winning eye tests without glasses

A two-part secret

The secret to winning eye tests without glasses has two parts. The first part is white, namely the 'Great White Glow' on page 146. The Glow appears when everyone uses their eyes the way nature intended: easily, without straining or trying.

Eyes see by receiving light from whatever you're looking at. A red ball sends only the red wave-length to the eye, absorbing all the other colours. White paper sends every colour to your eyes. Black print absorbs all the light, sending nothing to your eyes, therefore black letters are not actually seen. We recognise the shape of a letter by the white space around it. Teaching children early to mentally tune into the white spaces, rather than straining to see the 'unseeable' black print, will prevent many problems with reading books and eyecharts.

The second part of the secret is to finally recognise that eye tests are stress generators for children. Everyone should realise that eye tests are loaded with performance anxiety. This anxiety is akin to stage fright and in itself creates blur.

The unspoken obligation in eye tests

The pressure to see is not limited to letters on flat cards. There is an obligation charge on many things that appear in our visual field. Dr Bates observed that when people look at a plain white background their refractive error would lessen or disappear. When a child was being tested on an eye chart and other children were looking on, waiting to see what results Johnny came up with, Johnny went myopic. 'No child wants to be stupid,' said NVI teacher and optician, Helga Gryzb. She remembers her thought pattern from her first vision test at age six. In many children's minds, failing an eye test is equated with being stupid, a complete downer. Both myopic and hyperopic children register high on the obligation scale. High obligation creates stress, usually with great anticipation of failure thrown in.

High obligation	Low obligation
• black and white test charts	• plain white paper
• Mom's face when she's angry	• clouds, bunny rabbits
• jeering children's faces	• friendly glowing faces
• words in books	• sand on the beach

It is possible for all children to stay relaxed when reading letters in books and on eyecharts. Getting both side of the brain switched on helps; releasing test anxiety with Melting Beachballs does wonders. In this chapter you will learn a new method of relating visually to black and white print. Make this method, called Painting White, a life-long habit. See if any over-40s in your family will take off their reading glasses and join in.

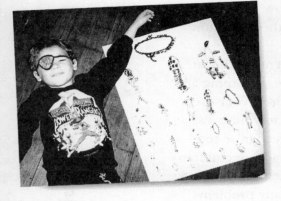

Daniel loves his viruses

Make your own eyecharts

My strategy for wringing the threat out of eye charts is to have NVI students make their own. In Vision Playcamps I ask the children what their favourite themes are. Ten year-old Anthony said soccer. Six year-olds Jack and Margo like cuddly animals. Daniel had just seen a TV program on viruses. Little Jack, at four, was enthralled with cars.

When the children were supplied with full-sized white poster paper and chunky black crayons, a collection of eyecharts appeared. Little Jack brought his collections of MotorCar magazines. He cut out cars and pasted them on the poster paper. The larger cars were at the top, diminishing in size to the bottom row. Even though some of the cars were coloured, Jack could still paint white around them, calling off their names from greater and greater distances.

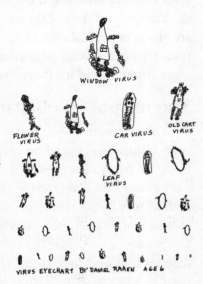

The viruses made small

144

After making a few theme eyecharts, we move to letters and numerals.

Have your child make her favourite letters on white paper with large black crayons or broad, felt-tip pens. Make letters in different sizes.

G H Z
Q X O

Cut the letters out and paste them on a piece of white poster paper. Hang your child's personal eye charts on the wall in the kitchen or in her room.

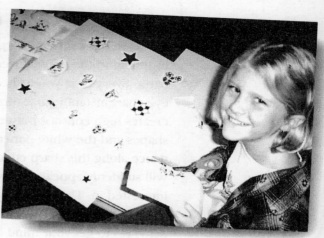

Mereki making her distance chart

You will end up with three different charts. The first one will have only shapes on it in the child's current and favourite theme. The next chart could have a mix of shapes and letters or words. The third kind she will be faced with on school eye-testing day or at the optometrist's office. The chart with only letters on it comes last. Do not worry about her memorising her charts; she will. Holding the familiar shapes in her mind and seeing them from farther away will build her confidence. When you begin Painting White games, sit at a distance from the chart where the top three lines are easy to recognise.

Shapes and letters eyechart

So far I have talked about eyecharts for distance blur. Children with high degrees of myopia, hyperopia or astigmatism may have blur at all distances. Hyperopes and astigmatics will need a small chart to hold in the hand with progressively smaller images. A myopic child with over four diopters of correction will also need a near point eye chart. In some cases you will be able to use a photocopier that reduces images to make the small chart. Or you can use a fine felt-tip pen and draw the progressively smaller hand cards. The goat and giraffe chart is from the Corbett school.

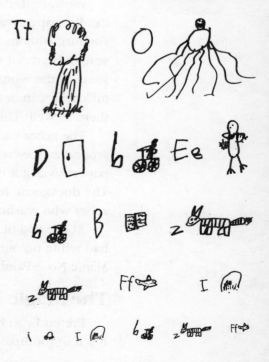

The Great White Glow

Since our eyes don't register black ink, we want to tune into the white spaces around the letters as a habit. Every time you glance at a black and white eye chart instantly go for the white spaces. This creates high contrast between the edges of the black shapes and the white paper. Your eyes will happily dance along this sharp edge. A brilliant white glow will suddenly appear around the shape you are interested in. This is the appearance of the Great White Glow. Do the following activities to get your mind acquainted with the Great White Glow. Once the Great White Glow has shown up, repeat the games to reinforce the friendship.

A White Thing

Begin by asking children what's white. Make a list of the answers. Do this while everyone is Palming. Put the white things together with action words.

For example, I asked a five year-old 'what's white'? Together we wrote down the following list:

snow, bird, daisy, dress, cloud, milk, doily, teeth, hair, shoes, candle, paper, waves, ice, polar bears, igloo, cream, ice-cream, yoghurt, ribbons, whiskers, wool goats, dove, goose, duck, pen, baby seal, in between the zebra stripes, egg, horse, socks. We then glued some of the words together obtaining zebrastripes, clouddress, milkdoily, candleteeth, creamgoose. Somehow stinkysocks got in there as well! Then we put together a little story:

The zebra had candleteeth and stinkysocks chasing a snowhorse around an ice-creamigloo. The babyseal cried icetears and the paperwaves got real big. The ice-creamigloo melted and floated away. The duckgoose fell in the yoghurt ocean and the daisybird sat on the zebra who washed his stinkysocks in the ice-cream.

At the end of conjuring up all these white pictures we definitely had white on our mind. Then we took the next step and imagined a Magic Nose Paintbrush.

The Magic Nose Paintbrush

Pretend you have a paintbrush on the end of your nose. You can dip it in toothpaste or shaving cream and paint everything you see

146

white . Paint the trees white, the people white, your toes white. Now let's paint white circles around the black animals and objects on the chart. Notice how the paper gets a white glow at the edges of the black. Let's close our eyes and imagine some fresh white paint on our brush. Got it? Now open your eyes and paint around the birthday cake at the top. A white glow, or aura, will appear around the birthday cake. Find more birthday cakes that glow. When surrounded by your white paint, the black shapes will become blacker. When the white is whiter and the black is blacker, you see the objects more clearly. The Great White Glow is here!

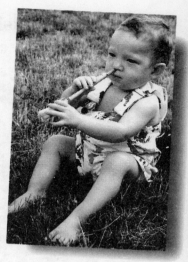

Aerro with his Magic Paintbrush

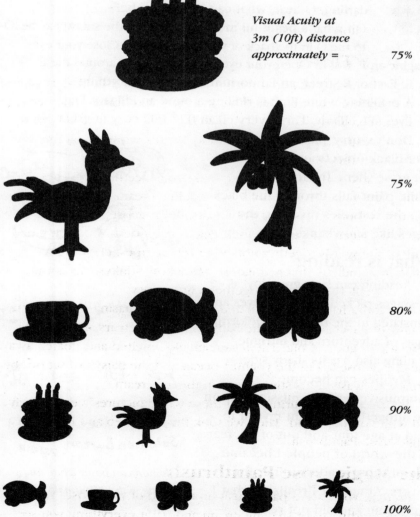

Visual Acuity at 3m (10ft) distance approximately =　　75%

75%

80%

90%

100%

Fishing and Finding

Rather than having your child look at blurry letters and then try to tell you what they are, let her find the letter shapes in her brain first with eyes closed, then paint white all over the chart with eyes open until that letter or shape jumps out at her. Whimsy helps banish the obligation factor. Encourage free association with the letters on the chart.

For example, the chart that Felicity is using has an 'O' and an 'E' on it. 'Close your eyes. Imagine an O. Got it? Open your eyes and paint white around the O.

O: Oh what a beautiful round donut. Become the 'O', scan, swing it around Odel Odel Ehihu.

CheeriOs, OKs, UFOs, O my, O gosh, O Goodness, O my darling, O dear, what can the matter be?

Oh what a beautiful mOrning. An O in the snOw. Say hellO to the O in the back of yOur nOse. Oink. Close your eyes.

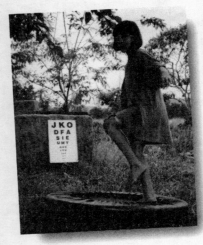

Felicity does Cross-Crawl, Paints White and goes whimsical with her eyechart

Imagine an E. Got it? Open your eyes and paint white around the E!

E: East of E Street, an Emporium that sElls EvErything.

A prEEning white Emu is rEEling around an ElEgant Egg.

Eyes sEE clEarly. ThrEE vEry clEan fEEt fEEl cosy in grEEn socks.

Don't worry, painting white over black objects and letters does not erase them. In fact a lot of white paint falls through the black ink, the rest piles up along the edges like snowbanks.

What is reading?

Reading can be a great joy, as messages picked up by the eyes are translated in the brain into colorful sagas of adventure and intrigue. Reading also has its shady side.

Myopes can become compulsive readers, missing out on life altogether. I taught myself to read at age four and out of my fear of the world of people I became one of those readers under the covers. At age 24 I realised what I was doing and did not read

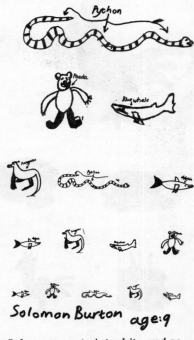

Solomon can paint white and go Fishing with his animals and their names

148 👁 Help Your Child to Perfect Eyesight

anything for a year. I had to pull myself away from the print on cereal boxes and newspaper headlines. Old habits. Now my life is too full to be satisfied with surrogate adventures.

Hyperopes can end up avoiding reading like the plague. Unpleasant experiences with reading in school, having to read in front of remorseless children, results in permanent allergic reaction to the printed word! Neither of these has to happen with our children if we can take a whole-brain, full-being approach to reading.

When reading, your eyes dance along the words in the pattern seen at the right.

Eye muscles must be fully relaxed to allow this rapid movement and clear foveal vision. The right brain sends in a message of mobility and release to the eye muscles. The left brain is consciously aware of the meanings of the words. The memory aspect of reading is both short and long term. Can you tell me what you just read? Could you tell me next week, without peeking at this page? If you could, then you have put this message into your right brain by translating the words into images.

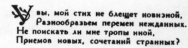

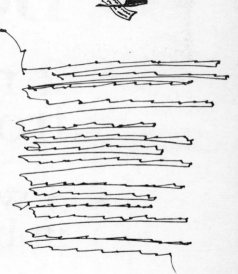

Record of eye movements while reading a Shakespeare sonnet (in Russian)

Paint White

Relaxed reading with understanding and memory can be accomplished with the use of the Magic Paintbrush.

Put your Paintbrush on the end of your nose and Paint White from left to right, through line one on page 150. Paint right over the black words which will reassert themselves. Blink easily, breathe, and go on with your Paintbrush through the second

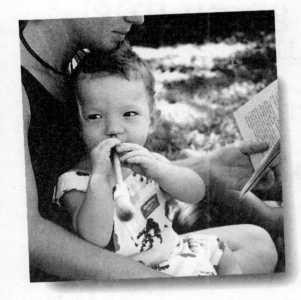

Carina uses an imaginary paintbrush, while Aerro practises

line . Let the Great White Glow appear. Continue to the bottom. After you have practised with this story, get one of your favourite books and practise painting with your Magic Nose Paintbrush through every line.

1 Geminy Boots

2 ran home from school

3 with a green frog in his hand

4 His father said to him

5 put that frog back in the pond

6 Geminy Boots ran in the rain

7 His frog never left him

8 It even slept in his bed

9 and ate oats for breakfast

👁 Help Your Child to Perfect Eyesight

The Geminy Boots story can be used to assess near point vision. If you read line 9 holding the page about 36 cm (14 in) away from your eyes, you have 6/6, 20/20, 100 percent close vision. Reading line number 8 means you have 6/12, 20/40, 80 percent close vision, adequate for Transition Glasses.

Learn this song to saturate your mind with whiteness. Music will help you keep white in mind while reading all books, papers and eyecharts.

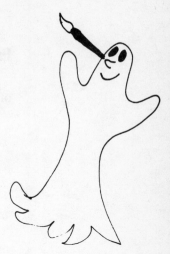

I Like Painting White

Words and Music by Donald Woodward

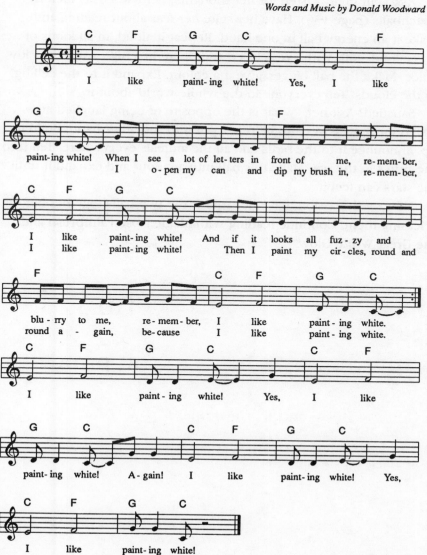

Emotions And Reading

Some thoughts and fears around reading alone, or aloud in front of others are:

I will get laughed at

I will sound funny

I will not be able to keep up with the other kids

I am stupid

My eyes hurt

I can't breathe

I won't understand the words

Ask your child. Listen for her thoughts, her fears. Play Melting Beachballs (page 136). Have her state her fear about reading and make it an energy ball in one hand. Repeat it aloud, in all kinds of ways: loud, soft, with eyes closed and open, in a high voice, in a low voice. Make the ball bigger, give it a colour. Expand it to the ceiling, to the clouds. Tell everyone in the whole world about it.

Satisfied? Ask her, 'What is the opposite of being laughed at?' Listen for the answer and help her put it in the other hand. Build it up, announce it to the birds and all the animals everywhere. Tell it to the fishes in the sea. Make this ball into a colour and expand it until the stars can feel it.

Now, with passion, have her squish the two balls together before releasing them. Continue reading with Magic Nose Paintbrush and the Great White Glow.

Part Three

Specific programmes for specific problems

Chapter Thirteen

Myopia

What is myopia?

When a child is myopic he will have blur in the distance and clear vision up close. If the myopia is severe he may have to hold objects within centimetres of his nose to see them clearly. In Australia this child is called short-sighted; in America he is called near-sighted.

The only representation of myopia found in school textbooks and popular magazines is an elongated eyeball. The abnormal length of a myopic eyeball drops the light beams from what you are looking at onto a point in front of the macula lutea. This means no clear central vision; no sharp edges on objects far away.

When the eyeball is too long, the image falls in front of the retina

One millimetre of elongation of the optical axis of the eye produces three diopters of myopia.

Pseudo or false myopia is also known. One awakens seeing the sign at the corner clearly. After a day at work, the sign is blurry. Direct explanations for pseudo myopia are scarce, but fatigue is a factor.

My high school biology book did not address the question of how eyeballs get too long. It simply shows a minus, concave lens placed in front of this strange organ. I wondered, 'If eyeballs can get longer, why can't they get shorter?'

They can - if visual habits are changed.

When does it start?

For many years myopic careers were started at age seven. More girls than boys became myopic at adolescence. By the time these children were eighteen, their myopia levelled off and stayed the same the rest of their lives.

A concave lens corrects for an eyeball that is too long.

This pattern has changed. Nowadays people at age 24 produce myopia for the first time; often at university or with a new job in a bank.

Some folks love the idea of teaching their children to read in the cradle. It's an enticing notion because precocious children are

 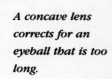

greatly admired, but some of these children become myopic at age four. A few mothers who have diligently home-schooled their bespectacled offspring glower at me resentfully when I mention a possible link between infants' reading and refractive error. I love the idea of home schooling. But if left-brain training is taking place that early, it needs balancing with right-brain vision games; and plenty of them. I used to think it would be great to have a seven year-old graduate from high school; my values have shifted.

What can we do for the child of seven or ten who is already dependent on glasses? Lots. With myopia it's not enough to throw glasses away. Vision games need to be played and inner feelings addressed.

If your myopic child is using a low prescription, (under two diopters), it may be possible to park his glasses in a drawer. If he is dependent on artificial correction to see the board at school, Transition or T-Glasses are called for.

Transition Glasses for young myopes

Your goal is to allow your child's vision to improve through the activities in this book while periodically stepping down the power of his glasses. Myopes, when they are not using lenses, experience **flashes** of clear sight. At first flashes last half a second, then for longer periods. A 12 year-old NVI student whispered to me after her vision class, 'My mum wanted me to tell you that I had a six hour flash.' I thanked her for telling me.

Most myopes can read easily without glasses unless they have significant astigmatism. Why then do myopes read with their specs? It is both from habit and because they have been told to.

For the purposes of this program we want children to be without glasses as much as possible so that the vision games can take effect. When they do need to set spectacles upon their noses, let it be with a minimum prescription. General guidelines for T-Glasses that you can take to your practitioner are on page 45. Pin-holes can also be used as T-Glasses for myopic vision.

If your child's prescription is below two diopters (my last pair of transition glasses for myopia were three and a half diopters), send a note to school asking all teachers to allow this child to sit in the front row. Give a copy of this book to his teacher. Vision games that help myopia also boost learning. Relaxed humans learn quickly.

With the requested strength of correction in the T-Glasses, your myopic child should be able to identify the letters and shapes on the next page from a distance of six metres (20 ft).

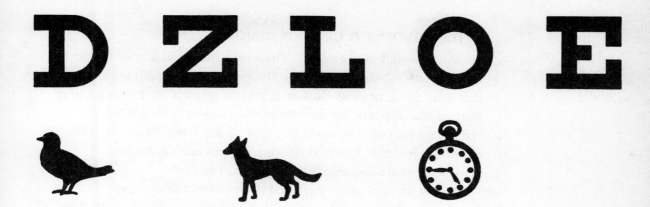

Think twice about surgery

Relatives who read the newspaper said to myopic Michael, 'Why go to that course? Just get yourself a 16-second operation and you'll see well enough.' Radial Keratotomy (Radial-K, or RK) will grow in popularity in the next decades. You could wait until your young myope turns 18 and send him to an ophthalmic surgeon.

An advertisement in a San Francisco subway asked: 'Would you like to wake up in the morning with 20/20 vision?' Yes, of course, but where is the small print? I collect it on RK. In 1985, writers of the Harvard Medical School Health Letter shifted their position on RK from guarded optimism to guarded pessimism. 'Between one and four years after the operation, only six percent of the treated eyes retained the correction achieved by the operation.' In 1988 Consumer Report magazine told us the US Air Force will not accept anyone who had undergone the operation. 'Many of the patients are bothered by glare at night and experience some fluctuations in their visual acuity.'

Techniques improve for shortening the myopic eyeball. Currently you can have epithelia (skin cells) blazed off the front of your eyeball by laser. Problems still remain. It takes four to five years for the cornea to heal fully; during this time the eyes are subject to infections. Sixteen percent of the eyes operated upon end up hyperopic; they over-react. Dr Walter Stark, director of corneal services at John Hopkins School of Medicine stated, 'Only a handful of ophthalmologists out of 13 000 have had the operation on themselves. If it were a simple cure-all as advertised, more would have had it.... You're talking about operating on a structurally normal eye with an unpredictable outcome.'

Radial keratotomy does not touch the **cause** of myopia.

What myopia feels like inside

Myopes walk on eggshells. Their sensitivity and fear of failure is frosted with capability illusions. Myopes become tough guys, debonair devils or class clowns. If you do scratch the frosting and a state of fear appears, do not attempt to console a myope by reminding him of how many trophies he has hanging on the wall. His distress is internal. External ribbons, badges and certificates of achievement are impressive, but they do not heal.

Young myopes feel compelled to be perfect in the eyes of others. But they remain imperfect in their own eyes. The way to help these children transmute their internal pressure is to do Emotional Healing on the issue.

Emotional Healing for myopia

Sit down together in a quiet place where you will not be disturbed. Use the following thought patterns to start inflating Melting Beachballs (page 136). After a bit of practice your child will begin to present his own findings, the launching pads for his emotional rockets.

Nobody loves me	Everybody loves me. I love myself
Everything I do must be perfect	I am loved even when I screw up
I hate making mistakes	I love making mistakes

You and your child put the sentence 'nobody loves me' in your right hands. As you repeat the phrase let memories and associations arise. Talk about it. Keep building up the size, colour and weight of the energy beachball in your right hand. Thoroughly explore the reality of this phrase, of this belief (even if adults try to deny it) until you are totally satisfied that you have told the wind and the world about it, that it is OK that nobody loves you because you can still love yourself (this is the secret ingredient).

Go to the opposite thought: 'Everybody loves me'. Somehow this is also true. Even the bully at school loves you, so does the girl who always whispers behind your back. Put the words, the thought, the feeling 'everybody loves me' in your left hand Beachball. Build it up to the stars, trumpet it through the galaxy. When you are satisfied with both your Beachballs, when they are somehow equal to one another, thunder-clap them together. Lightning flashes; the whole issue flutters away.

The myopia/hyperopia connection

These two visual conditions are like brother and sister: masculine and feminine aspects of sight. As your child is growing it is completely

158

natural for his vision to fluctuate between myopia and hyperopia.

Gesell's researchers peered into infants' eyes with a retinoscope from one metre away. I am paraphrasing Gesell's report and conclusions.

> 'A rattle was waved at 15 feet. As the four month-old child's eyes sought the noisy visual target, his eyes brightened and showed a myopic response. When his attention settled and held to the rattle, his eyes went hyperopic. As his attention relaxed, there was an oscillation between myopic and hyperopic response.

> 'The eye, like the hand is an organ of manipulation, and both are governed by the cortical brain. In the last analysis it is the brain which appropriates the outer world whether manually, orally, or ocularly. It does so by a projectile process, but this is a two-way reciprocating process - a directional process which emanates from within the self, goes out, and then returns within. The taking in and giving out process has a direct correlation to hyperopic and myopic states.

> 'When the child is older, his near visual tasks become more symbolic, but the retinal manifestations and the cortical (brain) demands are not profoundly different. The eye still functions as a prehensory and manipulatory organ. The preschool child's identification of a picture or a letter in a book is comparable to the infant's (grasping) and manipulation of a toy. The preschool child of three years looks for a familiar picture and since he knows what he is looking for, the retinoscope shows a sustained (myopic state). The organism is 'taking in' something — a visual kind of interjection. Presently the child extends arm and index finger and points to the picture; thereby he moves into the reciprocal outgoing phase of a circular cycle of response. Having 'taken in', he is now projecting externally...the retinoscope shows a shift toward hyperopia.'

Myopes and hyperopes reflect right- and left-brain imbalances, and they create distinct personality traits.

Myopes know a lot. They inhibit their impulses. They project inward rather than outward. Help young myopes unfreeze, expand, release themselves to love and imperfection.

Because myopia and hyperopia are two sides of the same coin, I suggest you read the following chapter on hyperopia. I emphasise close-to-far games in this chapter for myopes to help them take relaxation into the distance but do feel free to use games from the following chapter for your myopic child.

Reversing myopia with NVI

A note to parents

Even though all vision games are useful for myopia, emphasise the following: *'You' refers to the child.*

Cross-Crawl dancing

Switch on your right-brain for your eyes. Yes, it may already be switched on for your mind and body. We need it 'on' for your visual system (pages 84-85).

The Magic Nose Pencil

A Magic Pencil is essential for changing the myopic stare back into fast and loose saccadic movement (page 96). 'Penciling' becomes your new habit and you do it while watching TV, using your computer, all the time - including when you're using T-Glasses.

Palming

Palm whenever your eyes feel tired: go see the movies in your head. Palm when you wake up in the morning, just before sleeping, at your desk. Make what you have just read into images for long-term memory. Then facts will stick in your brain like peanut butter to the roof of your mouth.

Sunning

Sun once a day or whenever you can sneak it in. Sunglasses are not that cool, high light tolerance is (page 116).

Great White Glow

To see eye charts clearly as well as the board at school and the score at the football game, do Painting White with the Great White Glow at least twice a week (pages 146-148).

When reading books, make sure you sweep through the lines on the page with your White Paintbrush. Blink and yawn while reading. Do the same when you are planted in front of a computer (pages 149-151).

The Fishing Rod Story

Palm while listening to the following story. Paint the images that arise in your mind with your Magic Nose Paintbrush. This tale will help extend your clear vision into the far distance.

Lake Eyre is a huge, dry salt lake in South Australia. Every twenty years it fills with water after heavy rains. Thousands of pelicans and other birds go there to feed. After a few days the lake is dry again.

Derjundi is an Aboriginal boy who lives near Lake Eyre. He wrote letters to his pen pal Dennis who lives in Minnesota in North America. Minnesota is called the land of lakes. Dennis had caught the biggest rainbow trout of the year. He sent a photo of himself sitting in his rowboat, surrounded by fishing tackle and grinning from ear to ear. For Derjundi's tenth birthday, Dennis's family bought a shiny aluminum fishing pole with reel, wrapped it carefully and sent it by post to Australia. When the long cardboard box arrived at Derjundi's home in the desert four months later, his brothers and sisters jumped up and down with excitement.

The first thing Derjundi saw inside the box was green wrapping-paper covered with pictures of leaping trout. 'That's not the present,' he announced and ripped the paper off to reveal a glistening fishing pole. It had racing stripes painted on the rod and a cork handle. A fat reel of nylon fishing line and three large metal hooks fell out of the box. 'Whatever can you do with that?' wondered Derjundi's sisters and brothers.

'They must have thought you live by a lake with water in it,' yelled his little brother.

Derjundi shook his head. His father took the green paper and studied the pictures of rainbow trout.

After the flat horizon of Lake Eyre sliced the evening sun and ate it like toast, Derjundi walked out of his house with his fishing rod in hand. Kneeling in the crunchy sand, Derjundi carefully put the three lengths of the rod together. He wound the nylon line into the reel, just as it showed in the instruction book. He fastened a hook to the end of the line and sat down at the edge of Lake Eyre, waiting. His sisters and brothers ran home past him, laughing and pointing.

'He's going to catch a lot of dust devils and willy-willies.'

Derjundi sat quietly for a long time, swinging his head back and forth across the millions of stars in the clear, black sky. He stood up, flung his arm back and cast his fishing line into the sky. He heard the nylon line sizzle as it shot straight out from his fishing pole into the night sky. The sound stopped. Derjundi tugged on his rod. The line was stuck; Derjundi tugged harder and harder. He realised he had to turn the handle on the reel. He turned it and turned it more. The line moved and slid back onto the reel. Far off in the distance Derjundi could see something wriggling on the end of his line. It was silver and shiny like a popper from a metal soft-drink can. 'I must keep reeling it in,' he thought. The silver, wriggly thing finally lay at Derjundi's feet dangling from the end of his fishing line. He edged it with his Magic Nose Pencil and blinked at it and closed his eyes to remember if he had ever seen anything like it before. He had never seen anything exactly like this. He opened his eyes and whispered, 'You're a star.'

With the star safe inside his fishing bag, Derjundi jogged back home. He let his brothers and sisters and cousins have a peek at the star inside his bag. 'Tomorrow night I'll catch a supernova,' he announced to everyone.

Timetable for myopia games

birth to one year
    Rocking and Swinging, Massage and Point-Holding
one to three+ years
    Cross-Crawl Dancing
three to five+ years
    Palming and Near-Far Swings
five to ten+ years
    Magic Nose Pencil, Palming, Painting White and the Great White Glow, Nuclear Vision games and Painting Pictures

Chapter Fourteen

Hyperopia

What is hyperopia?

An eyeball that is too short is hyperopic. Blur results when viewing close objects. The short axial length of the eyeball causes the light beams from what you are looking at to fall behind the retina. A person could be so hyperopic that their blur range extends from up close into the landscape. The physical aspect of hyperopia is compensated for by placing magnifying (plus) lenses in front of the eye.

At birth most infants' eyes are hyperopic. By adolescence these short eyeballs should stabilise at the normal axial length creating a state called emmetropia, which means normal vision. For this reason, eye doctors tell parents, 'She may outgrow it. But have her wear these glasses in the meantime when she is reading.'

This approach encourages parents to put hyperopic children in glasses and wait to see what happens. Duke-Elder states that 50 percent of hyperopic children do in fact grow out of the condition; the other half end up as hyperopic adults in magnifying lenses.

The shortened eyeball lets the image fall behind the retina

Many children outgrow it

Optical professionals who find hyperopia with retinoscopy will recommend plus lenses for the child even when she can see clearly at all distances. Parents wonder why she should use glasses when she has no trouble seeing. The reasoning goes like this: accommodation is the ability of the lens of the eye to change its curvature. When you look at a tree on the far hill, your lens flattens. Glancing at the time on your watch causes ocular muscles to tighten and the lens to bulge, gathering in the light from your watch face to place it onto your macula lutea. If a child has strong lens accommodation (and most children do), she will be able to use this ability to focus on everything clearly, including her book.

A convex lens compensates for an eyeball that is too short.

For this reason, when asked, 'Why should she wear spectacles?', the optical specialist replies, 'Because she is using her accommodation ability to compensate for her too-short eyeballs. And if she does not use the magnifying lens I'm prescribing for her, her eyes are going to get very sore and tired from over-accommodating.'

I would rather give this child relaxation tools; Palming for tired eyes, and Painting White for effortless reading. My experience with hyperopic adults and children has shown that hyperopia is easy to dissolve with Natural Vision Improvement when the student is willing.

What hyperopia feels like inside

Hyperopic children are often wild cards, tantrum throwers, cross-eyed little demons, awkward misfits. In a recent Playcamp, five myopic instructors were matched to five hyperopic children. Two 1.8 metre (6 ft) male teachers had to forsake their carefully laid activity plans. The wee hyperopes were moving too fast. Not all hyperopic children bring pandemonium in their wake. Some are petite feminine dictators who run the show disguised as fairy princesses.

Hyperopic children are teachers come to jolt adults out of their conventions, out of their pedestrian trance. They are usually misunderstood. Their fantasies and insights have no precedent; teachers can't find their responses in textbooks. They must be wrong. Some hyperopes learn quickly and early to keep their right-brain antics well under control. Others blow you away with their explosions, demands and insights. I think these children contain yet-to-be-discovered solutions to world problems.

Hyperopes react to school desks like tigers to cages. **Why can't she sit still?** Even if the tiger is externally calm, an inner revolt is simmering. Anger is swallowed to cope with society. When grown-up, this girl may become an over-directive and strict music teacher.

Many hyperopes are on watch, playing eternal guard duty. NVI teacher Gloria Veit writes about her hyperopic childhood:

'It's possible that myopes are church mice with squeaky voices. That does not mean that I, as a hyperope, feel like a cat stalking those mice to eat them up. I feel more like the dog that looks after everything and everybody; making sure that no strangers get too close. I actually guard the church mice. Sometimes while playing with a delicate mouse my paws come down too heavily on her tail.

'If I look around and see any injustice being done I

will howl. If anyone tries to cage me, I will bite hard. I'm the fighter, the controller and the captain. I want to guard the world so it doesn't dissolve in chaos. Otherwise all the details will fly at me, penetrate my protective distance, pushy and invasive. Pushiness is something hyperopes can't stand. If someone comes too close to me I can't breathe.

'I assume that every hyperope carries around a secret wound, a basic fear of love. As a tiny child I felt that if I gave myself completely to love, someone would destroy it, the most precious thing in my life. So I decided to bury this precious jewel deep inside myself, so deep I forgot where it was. I'd be afraid to dig it out anyway. I convinced myself that people who love completely abandon themselves to pain. Anger is stuck in me. I'm stuck in anger. I was bitterly, angrily disappointed as a child when my love was rejected. Suppressing this anger made me strong, gave me a defence against the encroachment of others, and kept me from having to resurrect my love.'

(Translated from German by Janet Goodrich)

Emotional Healing for hyperopia

The hyperopic child is missing self love and refuses to get close to others or herself. This tendency lasts into adulthood. Hyperopic adults who search within find a small child who's angry at the world. She tells everyone to bug off and leave her alone. But this is not really what she wants. Her life energy pushes her to seek tumultuous and awkward contact. Use Melting Beachballs (page 136).

The general thought patterns of our small hyperopic friends

Go away	Come close to me
Don't look at me	Look at me
I want to disappear	I want to be here
I'm not here	I am here

Sit down comfortably together in a quiet place. Use these thought patterns to start with or listen for one the child may present herself.

Put the words 'go away' in your right hand. As you repeat the phrase, let memories and associations arise. Talk about it. Keep building up the size and colour and weight of the energy Beachball in your right hand. Go to the opposite only when you have thoroughly explored the reality of this belief, only when you are totally satisfied that you have told the oceans and the dinosaurs, the sky and everybody in the universe about it — that it is OK that everyone goes away because you can still love yourself a little bit when you are alone and rejected.

'Come close to me.' It's OK that people are sometimes mean and hurtful. It's OK that sometimes they spit in your face and call you names. **It's OK because you can still love yourself when they do this. You can still love yourself when you are hurting.** Put 'Come close to me.' in your left hand Beachball. Build it up to the stars, tell the Creator and the Universe about it. Whisper it to the ants on the ground. Tell the baby birds in their nests. When you are satisfied with both your Beachballs and they are somehow equal to one another, smoosh them together with a bang or a tiny sizzle. The baby birds are chirping happily and you can see clearly up close.

Reversing hyperopia with NVI

All the basic vision games in Part Two are helpful for hyperopia. However I'd like you to emphasise:

- Cross-Crawl dancing to switch on the left side of the brain for your visual system.
- Movement. In general hyperopes need lots of swings, free-form dancing; whole body activities. Thoroughly absorb Chapter Eight. The Magic Nose Feather and the Birds of a Feather Swing become a way of life. Refer to Chapter 19 for setting up physical environments that encourage total body and eye coordination.
- Resting your the eyes by Palming and visualising miniature worlds with lots of intricate details. A useful picturebook for hyperopes ages three to ten is 'The Bad-Tempered Ladybird' by Eric Carle. The print goes from small to large and back again while the grouchy ladybird (ladybug) meets aphids and a whale.
- The Magic Paintbrush and Great White Glow for reading large to small print.

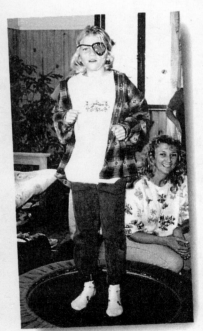

Mereki is hyperopic only in her right eye. Here she Patches, bounces and Paints White on her own eyechart

Shifting Images

Slide your Magic Nose Pencil from right to left on the following pictures. The little person or animal will shift from side to side in the opposite direction you are moving. This restores super fast saccadic motions. When you close your eyes and shift the images in your imagination, the effect is facinating.

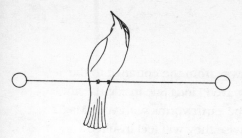

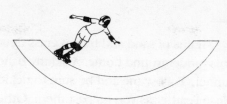

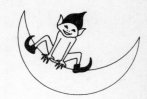

Light a candle and place it directly in front of you. Opening and closing your eyes, sweep to the right and the left of the candle. Notice how the candle moves in the opposite direction. Sing this song:

The Candle Swing

Words and Melody by Helen M. Kennedy

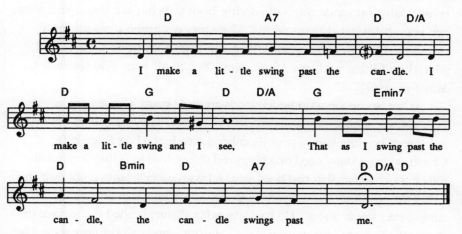

I make a lit-tle swing past the can-dle. I make a lit-tle swing and I see, That as I swing past the can-dle, the can-dle swings past me.

The Ant Queen

Hyperopes need to imagine small close shapes in their mind. Use the following story while Palming. Edge and tickle the tiny images with your Magic Nose Feather.

The Ant Queen

Linda Sue loved ants. She spent hours lying on her tummy watching ants collect food. As an experiment, Linda Sue put half her cheese sandwich on an ant path. In twenty minutes the sandwich had been pulled apart into crumbs and carried away to the ant nest. One day, while Linda Sue lay under a tree Palming she decided to go and meet the Ant Queen.

Making herself tiny with shrink dust from the supermarket, Linda Sue knocked on the door of Anthill Seventeen. 'Who's there?' demanded the ant who guarded the door. 'It's me — Linda Sue, Ant Lover. I'm wearing my black hat and my black coat and my black socks and I'm wearing my black sky-diving boots. Please let me come in. I want to visit your Queen and see all her tiny treasures.'

Grains of sand and bits of grass flew away from the entrance to the ants' underground home. A skinny hand waved Linda Sue inside the ant tunnel. 'Follow me and be sure to tickle the earthworms with your Magic Nose Feather as you go past them. Otherwise they will feel insulted.' Linda Sue followed the door-ant to a round room deep in the earth.

The Ant Queen, who was three times bigger than the humble door-ant, looked Linda Sue up and down with two emerald-green eyes. In her hand the Ant Queen held a white paintbrush. She was painting ant eggs.

'Ten thousand and twenty-three. That's enough for today,' sighed the Ant Queen. She put away her paintbrush, slopping a few drops of white paint on Linda Sue's skydiving boots. 'What are those and what are you and what do you want?' The Queen's green eyes glittered.

'Dear Queen, I'm an Ant Lover and I have come to OHHH and AHHH and Edge with my Magic Nose Pencil all your tiny treasures. May I please?'

'At last, someone who understands art and beauty. Come here, my dear. Edge these cunning, rare and priceless creatures.' The Ant Queen opened a jade green box the size of your thumbnail. Inside the box three baby Christmas bugs slumbered on cherry-red velvet. To Linda they looked like infant cockroaches that had been sprayed with metallic auto paint. But she didn't say anything. 'Now I will show you something that no one up top should ever know about.' 'Up top' was what the ants called the surface of the earth. The Ant Queen tugged on a ring attached to a flat grey rock. The rock lifted; dust flew in all directions. A hundred gold eyes gleamed out of the dark hole. The Ant Queen scooped up one of the 'eyes' and laid it in Linda Sue's hand as she whispered, 'This is left over from our visit with the Spanish Conquistadores.' Linda Sue traced the round edges of a gold coin with her Magic Nose Pencil. She noticed faint lines scratched on its surface. She swept the coin with a delicate gold-coloured Magic Nose Feather and read the words, 'Love is everywhere. Alphonso Saltamontes 1492'.

What other tiny objects could the Ant Queen show Linda Sue and Palming children in her treasure chamber? The first Ant Queen's baby rattle, the royal collection of matchbox cars, a fungus rock star in a jar and microbes playing tennis.

Now it's your turn to imagine more tiny, miniature, miniscule, microscopic, wee things.

The Swinging Ball

This game brings forth saccadic movement and quick identification of shapes. It releases high spirits. Use a lightweight ball that won't hurt anyone who gets in the way. Styrofoam works well. Invite myopes into the game to help them lose their stare.

In fabric and craft shops you will find inexpensive white Styrofoam balls of various sizes. In Playcamps we use large 15 cm (six in) balls. Students paint them with acrylic paints in bright colours. Each ball is painted all over in a solid background colour. When the background is dry, identifiable images are painted in contrasting colours e.g. stars, trees, cats, cars or dots.

With pliers make a small eye on a length of stiff wire 20 cm (8 in) long. Tie a one metre, (three ft) long string to the wire eyelet. Pierce a channel through the middle of the foam ball with the wire. Pull the string through at the same time. Untie the string from the eyelet. Fasten a button or bead to the string so it cannot pull back through the ball. Remove the wire from the ball and hang it from a high place where you can all lie in a circle underneath it. Keep the ball swinging. As you bat the ball, follow it with your nose. Blink and breathe. See if you are able to edge a star or cat while the ball is travelling.

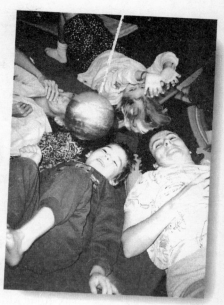

Daniel, Mereki, Soloman and their mothers keep the Swinging Ball moving

Timetable for hyperopia games

birth to two+ years
> Do the Baby Eaglet Swing
> Bounce on the mini-trampoline
> Have lots of crawling adventures

two to ten+ years
> Cross-Crawl dancing
> Palm for story telling with small and close images

four to ten+ years
> The Swinging Ball
> Bird of a Feather Swing
> Magic Nose Pencil
> Reading with the White Paintbrush
> Make and use your own black and white reading cards
> Resolve inner turmoil with the Melting Beachballs

Hyperopia is often accompanied by astigmatism and/or strabismus. If your child has a combination of these symptoms the following chapters will help. On special days you would add games to iron out astigmatism and re-direct eyes and brain toward fusion.

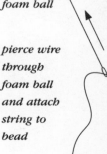

bead fastened to string

foam ball

pierce wire through foam ball and attach string to bead

Chapter Fifteen

Astigmatism

What is astigmatism?

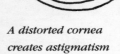

Astigmatism is usually a warp in the cornea at the front of the eye. It can also occur in the lens.

The visual effect is akin to looking through an old window pane that has waves in it or in a carnival mirror.

There are two kinds of astigmatism, regular and irregular. The regular kind occurs at a particular angle and can be corrected with a cylindrical lens ground into glasses or healed with NVI. Irregular astigmatism is usually due to a disease condition or accident. It cannot be satisfactorily corrected by glasses.

A distorted cornea creates astigmatism

How it feels and looks

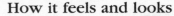

Astigmatism causes visual blur and tired eyes at all distances. Even a slight amount can result in aching, scratchy eyes after reading for five minutes. Distortion in the distance can be unnoticeable until you have to read a street sign. If

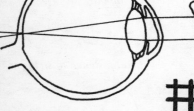

A cylindrical lens corrects for astigmatism

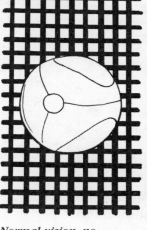

Normal vision, no astigmatism

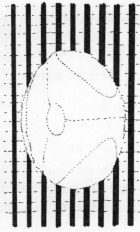

This figure shows horizontal astigmatism. It is corrected by a cylindrical lens at axis 180 degrees.

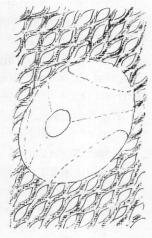

Here oblique astigmatism blurs everything at 45 degrees. It is corrected by a cylindrical lens at 45 degrees.

the warp is vertical all the upright letters such as E, P, B, T and L, will be blurred posts. If you have astigmatism at 60°, the Z in Zebra will be blurred.

The cause of astigmatism

In ophthalmic literature, astigmatism is blamed on the upper eyelid pressing on the cornea. Dr Duke-Elder states that 68 percent of children at the age of four and 95 percent at the age of seven have this kind of astigmatism. When the child grows older, pressure astigmatism tends to disappear or reverse itself into the opposite angle.

You can produce astigmatism easily for yourself right now by pressing your finger against your eyelid or 'by the action of the extra-ocular muscles,' as Duke-Elder writes. The extra-ocular muscles are those six big muscles (page 95) which rotate and move the eyeball in all directions. Could a pair of muscles be holding tight?

A cylindrical lens is placed in glasses to compensate for astigmatism in the optical system of the eyes.

How correction is determined

Optometrists and ophthalmologists employ both mechanical and subjective means of determining the amount and angle of astigmatism correction. If a child is old enough to respond adequately, the doctor will try with the best of intentions to come up with an accurate prescription by placing a lens and a letter in front of the child's eyes. The question is asked, 'Is this better or is this better?' as the lenses are changed. As an astigmatic child I remember being confused and stressed by this questioning. I perspired in my effort to give that nice man the right answer.

It appears and disappears

Astigmatism distortion in the eyes and in the visual field can be here at one o'clock and gone at two o'clock. I had challenged my students many times in teacher training courses with this statement. Finally a certified teacher in Munich paid her money and visited three different optometrists in one afternoon. Sure enough, she came home with three different prescriptions. The amount of astigmatism changes. The angle shifts. If you yourself have old prescriptions for astigmatism in your drawer, take a look. Notice if strength and direction has changed.

60° astigmatism will do this to a "Z"

A cylindrical lens focuses a line to a point

A child's eyes will continually attempt to please a correction ground into his lenses. Doing the activities in this chapter will help smooth away astigmatism warp. If your child puts glasses back on with correction for astigmatism in them, his progress is wiped out.

If members of the optical industry find a trace of astigmatism during an eye exam, most of them will insist on putting correction for it into the child's glasses. Their motives are impeccable: 'He will get headaches and severe eyestrain if we do not correct for astigmatism.' They have the best of intentions and don't want anyone to suffer the pain of uncorrected astigmatism.

I speak from acute personal experience. My last pair of fully corrected lenses had five diopters of astigmatism correction for my right eye and two diopters for my left. Conscientious optometrists and medical doctors drew careful diagrams for me of the eyeball, sympathised with my inevitable reading distress, and insisted on a correction for astigmatism. I insisted back. In my first pair of T-Glasses the astigmatism was cut by half to two and one half diopters for my right eye. It was taken out completely on the left side.

In the guidelines for T-Glasses I say, 'Take out all astigmatism correction if possible.' In my case the warp on my right cornea was too great to immediately cut out all astigmatism correction. I needed some of it to see 6/12 through my driving glasses. Astigmatism correction may have to be juggled with myopic or hyperopic correction. You need an extremely cooperative practitioner, who understands that you will be playing 'erase astigmatism' games with your child. If your son needs to see the board at school it may be necessary to leave some astigmatism correction in his lenses; but I stipulate, with caution: if he has less than one diopter, leave it out.

An Astigmatism prescription

A prescription for astigmatism only, in one eye only, should look like this:

The word axis designates the angle of astigmatism. The cylindrical lens is ground in the glasses at the angle determined

	SPH (sphere)	CYL (cylinder)	AXIS
Right Eye		-1	x15
Left Eye			

by an optometrist or ophthalmologist.

Think about geometry. For example, if the axis number is 45, then a cylindrical lens is placed at 45° as you see on the figure at right.

👁 Help Your Child to Perfect Eyesight

Note: the word 'sphere' in the prescription example refers to a correction for either myopia (a minus '-' will appear before the number of diopters) or for hyperopia (a plus '+' will appear before the number of diopters). Astigmatism usually occurs in combination with myopia or hyperopia, rarely all by itself.

Erase astigmatism with NVI

Emphasise switching on the whole brain with Cross-Crawl Dancing. Do Bird of a Feather Swings. Using the Great White Glow and Magic Paintbrush when reading will minimise fatigue and blur.

The following games for astigmatism can be played in two ways. Sweeping along every angle will help saccadic movement and eye mobility in general. The game can be made more specific if you know the angle of astigmatism. You can then spend most of your time sweeping your Magic Nose Feather or Magic Paintbrush along that angle.

The angle and amount of astigmatism could be different in each eye. In this case, you can separate the eyes by using a Pirate Patch (see page 192.)

Zoo Train and Birds on a Wire

Guide your child through the following activity:

Zoo Train

With your Magic Nose Feather swing and sweep on the vertical part of the railway track for a few seconds.

Close your eyes and do exactly the same movement, keeping the image of the railway track in your mind.

Open your eyes again,

North East

South West

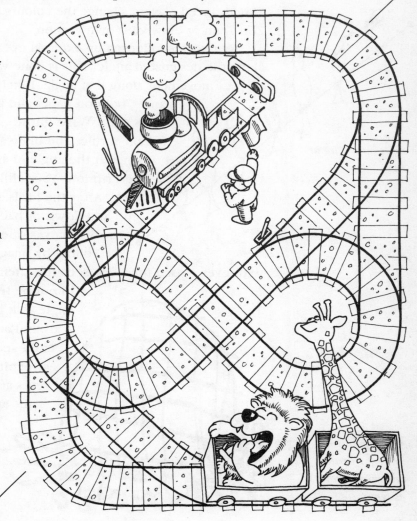

sweeping up and down the track. Repeat the same process with the horizontal railway track.

Do the same three-step process with the north-east and south-west tracks.

Imagine a train engine takes off around the figure eight track. Give it a colour. Pink with green smoke? Good. Close your eyes and imagine it's travelling around the whole track. Open again. After the train makes three complete revolutions around the track it picks up a freight car. The freight car is also pink. It contains a yawning lion. Follow the train around the track with engine and one lion car, eyes open, eyes closed. Attach another car. The second car contains a giraffe. Pink, of course. You can see its long neck sticking out. Round and round we go, eyes open for a while, then closed. You can add as many cars and animals as you like. This becomes a memory game. For advanced players, change the colours of the cars. Photocopy the Zoo Train or draw your own version.

Your goal is to loosen up external eye muscles that guide the eyes along the designated angle. This is done with right-brain imagery and movement along that angle. It helps to make your own visual games, both on paper and in the landscape.

Birds on a Wire game

Birds on a Wire at 135°

Take a ruler and draw a straight black line on paper at the angle of astigmatism shown on the prescription. Your child then draws birds on the 'wire'. After the birds are drawn, he then slides up and down or back and forth on that line with his eyes open for a few seconds.

Follow by imagining the Birds on a Wire with eyes closed for a few seconds, then again with eyes open.

(Do not be terribly precise about the angle as it is probably wriggling around anyway.) Make sure your child keeps his head level when sweeping along the wire so his eyes are saccadically vibrating at the appropriate angle. You can vary this game by asking your child for his favourite theme: draw a series of dinosaurs marching along the wire, cars, coins or

An astigmatism turtle for vertical and horizontal astigmatism

Help Your Child to Perfect Eyesight

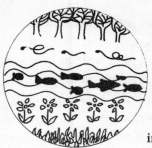

Plants and animals at 180°

soccer balls. Draw balloons, lollipops, or birds flying, animals, flowers, spider webs, spaceships or gold fish. Do it on paper, then imagine your goldfish are swimming on the wall; then across the sky.

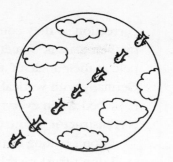

Goldfish at 45°

After swinging and sweeping along friendly images on paper, walls and skies, sing this song. Follow along all the lines you can find with your Magic Nose Pencil.

What astigmatism feels like inside

Astigmatic eyes ache. It is seeing at the emotional level of pain. The unconscious thought is 'it hurts to see.' This is evidenced by an indirect response in eye muscles, either the large outside muscles pulling across the cornea or the ciliary muscle tugging on the lens of the eye.

Lines, Straight Lines

Music - Traditional

Words by NVI Teacher Dede Callichy

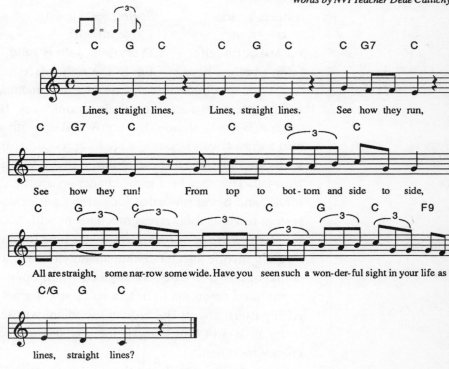

Astigmatism results in painful seeing at all distances. Reading makes sandpaper eyes. When looking into the distance there is a sensation of displacement. Even though the hills and buildings are upright, there's a warped feeling inside the mind.

Adult NVI students with a lot of astigmatism stopped using

correction so they could explore painful sensations previously blocked by their glasses. Sometimes they sat still, gazing steadily at a black line held at their angle of astigmatism. During this exercise a woman in Germany with vertical astigmatism recalled being left behind in her baby bed when everyone else ran to the bomb shelters. Tobias Mosner, NVI instructor, wrote down the thoughts that arose for him.

I don't belong in this world

I don't trust myself

I don't trust where I take myself with my own ideas

The astigmatism shift keeps me away from myself

Everything I do is wrong. Everyone else is right

Emotional Healing for astigmatism

Four main issues emerge as mental and emotional partners to astigmatism:

It hurts to see	Seeing feels good
I hate myself	I love myself
I mistrust myself	Everything I do is valid
I don't belong here	I'm in the right place

There are children who cannot abide making a mistake or getting anything less than an 'A' on their school work. Humiliation and internal burning shame that is covered up with a blanket or shoved into a drawer can become a life-long reaction. To ease this hidden stress we must teach these children that love is still here for people who fail. This may be a great challenge if your child is attending school and being rewarded for perfect performance. The school system rewards their stress mechanism with accolades.

Myopes are seeking approval and love from outside themselves. If a young myope also has astigmatism, you have a deluxe recipe for denial of life. Don't be too shocked when opening a box of suppressed emotions to hear a voice say, 'I want to die.' The death-wish pattern affects the kidney meridian, whose affirmation is 'I love being alive.' In Chinese medicine, eye disturbances are linked to the kidney meridian.

Let's deal first with the theme 'I hate myself.' It may be difficult to conceive that small children are already judging and rejecting themselves. Yet anyone who has worked with a child perfectionist or a child with learning difficulties knows that this theme of self-disapproval is constantly active, even at home and on the playground.

Use the Melting Beachballs (page 136)

Put 'I hate myself' in your right hand. Make it into an energy ball with colour and weight. Build it up while you repeat the words 'I hate myself'. Is it OK to hate yourself?

It's OK to hate myself, yes.

Is it OK to bring it out and say it aloud, even yell it to the treetops until it is somehow funny?

Next you ask for the opposite. Your child may have a different answer from 'I love myself'. Go with the child's truth.

'I love myself, I love myself.' Feel how the sound of these words vibrate in your body. If it's not true yet, then go right back to the opposite, until you can return and enjoy 'I love myself.'

OK. Under all circumstances, I can love myself, even when I don't know the answer to the maths problem; even when I say something stupid; even when I hurt someone else's feelings and need to apologize. It's OK to hate and to love myself.

Bring both Beachballs together like party balloons, like coloured foam, like... well, you tell me....

Other therapies

Astigmatism can be mechanically related to displaced skull bones. Contrary to popular belief, skull bones never completely fuse together. The eye socket is constructed of several moveable bones. These bones encasing the eyes and optic nerves can be manually adjusted. In children the skull is extremely flexible. Osteopathic textbooks show photographs of children's heads which had been distorted by difficult births: by forceps or suction delivery. In many cases adjustment of the skull bones resulted in improved sight as astigmatism disappeared. Some chiropractors are trained to perform adjustments to the skull. Look for an osteopath or chiropractor who does 'craniopathy'.

Chapter Sixteen

Strabismus and lazy eyes

What is strabismus?

An eye muscle that does not release or relax fully can hold an eye in a fixed position, away from the line of sight. This condition is called strabismus or *squint*, depending on how severe the turn may be. In this chapter I will use the word strabismus interchangeably with 'turned eye'.

The muscles of a turned eye are either not receiving correct messages from the brain or, if the message does come through, the muscles may be unable to respond because the bone to which they are attached to is tilted within the skull. When the brain says look

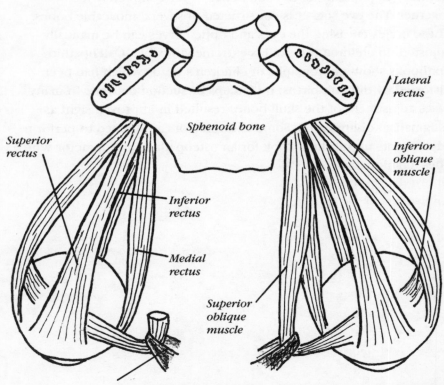

Eye muscles are directed from the brain and are attached to skull bones

Superior rectus

Sphenoid bone

Inferior rectus

Medial rectus

Lateral rectus

Inferior oblique muscle

Superior oblique muscle

Trochlea. The superior oblique muscle slides through this pulley.

👁 Help Your Child to Perfect Eyesight

straight ahead, or left or right, the pair of eye muscles which turn the eyes in the desired direction do not respond properly. One muscle remains cramped and its partner refuses to contract.

There is usually nothing wrong with the eyeball itself, unless squint has been started by a disease process. A turned eye can become a 'lazy eye' if the message from that eye is not used by the visual brain in the process of seeing.

This is what turned eyes look like from outside.

Alternating Squint means the child looks first with one eye, then the other. The 'switched off' eye usually goes inward.

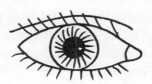
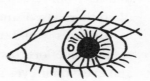

Exotropia means the eye turns outward (wall-eyed). The eye diverges

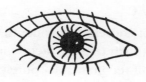
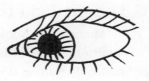

Esotropia means the eye turns inward (cross-eyed). The eye converges

Misalignment of eyes can occur in other directions as well. Even a slight deviation from ideal coordination results in fatigue and disturbance of some brain functions.

A turned eye signifies unbalanced brain activity. Human eyes are designed to work together, simultaneously pointing toward and saccadically vibrating around the same point in space. The organism must use 500 percent of body energy, instead of the usual 25 percent allocated to vision, to overcome misalignment. Ultimately, the brain decides to turn off the message from one eye, conserving energy for other duties. A 'lazy eye' results. The official term for lazy eye is amblyopia ex anopsia. If remedial action of some kind is taken, amblyopia can be avoided or reversed.

Why eyes turn

Medical information given to parents describes the crooked tree but not its roots. In 'The Well Baby Book', Dr Samuels explains, 'The eyes are not properly aligned due to unequal strength and faulty balance in the muscles surrounding the eye.' The next question hangs in the air: 'What causes unequal strength and muscular imbalance?'

Searching for the root cause of strabismus led me to dig deeper, via medical textbooks and phone calls to osteopaths and behavioural optometrists.

Cameron Dawson, of Dawson Technologies in Victoria, teaches therapists to correct strabismus by gentle manipulation of the cranial bones. Eye muscles attach to skull bones. 'In the majority of cases turned eyes result from the bones of the skull not being in the correct position.'

Behavioural optometrists sometimes blame turned eyes on environmental interferences during the binocular development stage. Richard Kavner OD, in his book 'Your Child's Vision', says head injuries from forceps deliveries are a cause. But he feels that most often there is a disturbance of the neural control centres in the brain.

Dr Bates would say that eyes are turning because the child is making an effort to see. When his small patients relaxed their minds and eyes, their eyes straightened.

Parents have a number of options to consider.

The medical response

Medical textbooks do not address in any depth emotional, mental, environmental or historical (birth trauma) factors in squint. Therefore medically trained doctors will recommend a purely physical approach, which, according to Duke-Elder, is:

A surgical plaster over the straight eye day and night for three months. 'The defective eye is thus coerced into activity.' The child must be checked by the MD during this period 'since the deviation sometimes becomes transferred to the occluded (covered) eye and the vision in it may deteriorate.'

Atropine drops may be given to the parents to place in the child's good eye. With atropine distance vision becomes blurred and near vision becomes impossible. Atropine is a drug which affects the autonomic nervous system.

From 'Mim's Manual': 'Atropine sulphate is widely used in ophthalmology as a powerful mydriatic and cycloplegic. Dilation of the pupil occurs within half an hour of its local application and lasts for a week or so. Atropine is used both pre-operatively and post-operatively in many types of intraocular surgery. It is also used in refractive work with children.'

In Australia, Atropine sulfate is listed as a S4 medicinal poison. The regulations regarding S4 poisons vary somewhat from state to state. For Western Australia we read:

> S4 to be labelled Caution, supply without prescription illegal: keep out of reach of children.
> Supply restricted to prescription or authorized person

👁 Help Your Child to Perfect Eyesight

with an allowance for some emergency supply for continuation of human therapy. Prescription to be cancelled unless repeated. Order validity 12 months. Advertising not permitted except in bona fide professional journals. Records of prescriptions dispensed to be maintained.

Duke-Elder states:

> 'The results of such treatment are very varying. If the eye were amblyopic (and turning) before treatment commenced, the good eye would be occluded for a month, and if no improvement occurs a further month may be tried. If this too proves fruitless, all hope of ultimate functional utility may be abandoned. If better vision can be elicited, occlusion should be continued. Provided the case is carefully supervised, there need be no hesitation in continuing this for considerable periods of time, as long as any improvement is obtained.'

At this point the surgeon may decide on *orthoptic* treatment; visual training for binocular vision. If orthoptic training does not work, the next step is surgically clipping the overtight muscle or resetting its attachment to the eyeball. This is done under general anaesthesia.

Language is a powerful tool. It can become a cattle prod when used by authority figures. If you feel threatened or intimidated by medical jargon or emotionally loaded words, admit it. This will allow you to avoid being goaded into actions you feel in your heart are wrong. 'Blind' is a particularly frightening term. 'Your child will go blind in that eye if she does not have an operation now.' Let's examine this message under a magnifying glass.

The word 'blind' used in this context signifies amblyopia. The eye is not blind in the usual sense. In fact if the 'good eye' were destroyed, the turning eye would come back on stage. In most cases the turned eye is physically healthy. This use of the word 'blind' is therefore highly misleading. Notice its effect in your nervous system and hesitate twice before making a decision out of panic.

What about the time pressure? If you wait any longer your child will go 'blind'. Pause at least long enough to consult with three unconnected medical specialists and with behavioural optometrists who work directly with strabismus. David Evian OD, who runs a clinic in Sydney for strabismus training, asserts, 'For every theory there is a counter theory.'

The 'closed window' theory says that if overtight muscles are not operated upon during a certain time in the child's brain development it is too late: the window slams shut. Does the window open and close between four and six months, between birth and age five, between ages four and ten? Or does it never close? The professionals have varying opinions.

You must operate on this baby with a turned eye before it is six months old. From studies covering the eyes of chicks and kittens it has been found that after this stage the cells in the visual cortex will no longer respond and the child will never get fusion. Operate now.

Children with squint must be operated on before the age of seven. After that they will not get fusion, nor will they be able to speak a foreign language without an accent, as the appropriate cells in the brain will not be willing to learn a new pattern.

This cross-eyed child must be operated on before the age of ten. After that the organism is too set in its ways.

Imagine a conference where ophthalmologists, perception psychologists, neurologists, paediatricians, behavioural optometrists, osteopaths and chiropractors got together to discuss the 'Closed Window' theory. Fur would fly.

Behavioural optometrists train turned eyes

The goal of ophthalmic surgery and orthoptics is fused binocular vision. Everyone doing vision training has this same goal, including optometrists and NVI teachers.

Behavioural optometrists use visual training with optical devices rather than surgery and drugs or surgery plus orthoptics. There are ten to 20 clinics in Australia where full training services are offered for children on a weekly basis. I spoke with Graeme Thompson, representative of the ACBO, Australasian College of Behavioural Optometrists in Sydney. He said, 'A lot of surgery is done but it is a cosmetic success. The eyes are straight, but the function is still strabismic. You can't gauge success by the appearance of the eyes.'

Dr Kavner states the case more strongly:

> 'A parent who seeks advice about a child's turned eye is frequently told that the only thing to do is to have ocular surgery. Not only is this advice incorrect and misleading, it can be dangerous in ways we hadn't thought of before. In fact, relatively few cases of strabismus are due to faulty muscles. Surgery may therefore be entirely unjustified in many cases.'

Every operation using anesthesia carries risk.

By 1978, eleven independent surveys assessing the success rate of orthoptics for strabismus had been made. The results varied from 34.2 percent to 92.7 percent. This data came from both optometric and ophthalmic sources. The two optometrists who collated the surveys concluded, 'Although the ophthalmological-orthoptist strabismus cure rates of 56 percent achieving high level functional cures and 67 percent achieving cosmetic success are impressive figures, the optometric studies show a high level functional cure rate of 76 percent and almost 86 percent cosmetic success. A "functional cure" means the children are achieving fusion. "Cosmetic success" tells you the eyes are straight, but the messages from the two eyes are not being used simultaneously by the visual brain.'

Cranial adjustments

For this book Cameron Dawson writes,

'Conventional anatomy teaches that the bones of the skull are separate at birth and become one solid static cranial structure in adult life. The baby's head needs to be very flexible at birth to fold the cranial plates gently, allowing access into the world through the birth canal. Every mother in the Western world is made aware of the fact that the open areas between the cranial plates, the fontanelles, are to be avoided to limit any damage to the baby's brain. This misinformation is the root cause of the problems of strabismus and learning difficulties. What mother indeed is going to allow any untoward pressure to her beautiful new baby's head, but this inhibits her taking the natural action that every other mammal mother takes in caressing by hand or tongue the head of the newborn. This attention by the mother is a natural instinct and places cranial plates back into correct position after they've been misaligned through the birth process. Fortunately statistics show that two out of three babies achieve the correct alignment of the head bones by chance and there is no further problem. It is the other 30-odd percent where problems arise.

'Balinese people follow an ancient practice derived from their Polynesian and Indian heritage. Babies are massaged at birth, both body and head for a moon and two days. The mother is taught this technique by her mother-in-law. Bodily massage continues in another form throughout the child's lifetime.'

In America, the home of cranial osteopathy, the skulls of newborns are checked by osteopathic physicians for birth trauma. Slight or gross damage to the skull can cause constant unexplained crying, breathing disorders, frequent infections, learning problems, astigmatism and strabismus. Like the Point Holding described in Chapter Six, remedial treatment is light, rhythmic and sustained until a change is detected.

In NVI seminars adults who had numerous operations as children and whose eyes still turned, were able to obtain fusion. This was accomplished with switching on the whole brain, with directional fusion games and with Emotional Healing. Every one of these people cried with joy when they looked in the mirror at two straight eyes, eyes that were ready to play fusion games. A man in Virginia, who had spent 20 years trying to get fusion, said orthoptists had thrown him out as a hopeless case. I suggested he remember a scene from his childhood, instead of trying to fuse with his left brain. He was instantly successful. A letter six months later reported that he still had fusion.

Your options
Wait and see; do nothing

This is not my style but I honour anyone's right to do this. A woman once said to me that she had healed her eyesight through prayer. I honour that approach too.

Take your child immediately to an ophthalmologist for a thorough exam, diagnosis and recommended medical treatment

I think it is a good idea to get an expert diagnosis. However, if seeking treatment I would certainly roam far and wide to find a person and a clinic where the treatment process does not traumatize the child. Surgical treatment is more readily available than anything else but it leaves a trail of shattered and frightened children who sometimes refuse any kind of help thereafter — even if it is NVI fun and games, mildly presented under a tree. When they hear the words eyes, fusion, doctor, clinic, some of these children freeze up or disappear out the door.

Seek examination and treatment with vision training from a behavioural optometrist

Behavioural optometrists are trained to thoroughly examine eyes and prescribe glasses and/or visual training for children with strabismus. Seek out someone who has an empathetic assistant who will serve as teacher and friend to the child. These sessions usually run for an hour once a week.

Search for and use natural therapies

Oh, for a Balinese mother-in-law, a skilled cranial osteopath or even a chiropractor trained in cranial adjustments! You may have to search high and low, or travel, but such rare birds do exist. In the meantime, use the vision games and the resources in this book.

Find yourself an NVI teacher or train to become one yourself

Please note that NVI is not a substitute for examination and diagnosis of eyes as we are not trained to do either of those. We are, however, prepared and educated to play vision games and do Emotional Healing with children in a human, informal fashion that can be used in conjunction with any of the above approaches, except the first one (see page 260).

Straighten turned eyes with NVI

The most important thing to remember when playing Natural Vision Improvement games with turning eyes is the concept of phoria. Phoria is Latin for tendency. It is used in the optical industry to designate the tendency of the line of vision to deviate from normal.

Favouring the phoria

This means inviting (rather than coercing) the turning eye to move in the desired direction. For example, if the right eye wants to stick to the nose then we wish to entice (not force) the right eye to look in an outward direction. Usually people say the eye must be made to work. Don't work an eye, muscle or brain that is already under stress. Let the eye and its muscles relax and play along with the child they belong to.

Principles to remember for favouring the phoria

Use the following ideas and vision games to coax and invite turned eyes in the direction they need to go.

Eyes are attracted to light and movement with

penlights	a ball on a string
candles	windchimes
glitter	bells & windmills

Eyes are attracted to colour and contrast. Use complimentary colours when making Tromboning Paddles (page 187).

black and white
blue and orange
red and green
yellow and violet

Contrary to assumption, tiny children do have long attention spans. When the entertainment is paced to the child's level and kept simple, she will extend the game and ask for repetition. Carina at nine months pulled a pair of underpants on and off her head 97 times. Aerro at 19 months performed an acrobatic somersault over my body twelve times in succession, applauding himself after each roll.

Games for babies with turned eyes (birth to one year) +

The Flying Spoon

Make eating into a phoria game. Get her attention with delicious food on a spoon. Bring the spoon toward her from the appropriate side. It can do some aeronautical tricks before it lands in her mouth.

Hang her batting mobiles so the kicking foot attracts her eye in the desired direction.

Play Tug-of-war. Lay baby on the floor. Let her tug on the towels.

Touch draws the attention of the eyes. If something crawls across your skin while you are lying outdoors under a tree, you jerk to attention and send your eyes in that direction, to identify the crawler as friend or foe. Should you kiss it or swat it?

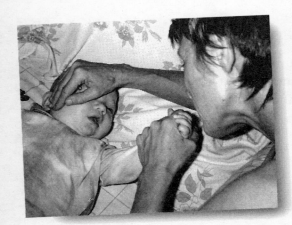

Gently covering the straight eye, talk to the turning eye

Most people instinctively use their fingers to draw an infant's attention. Notice from which direction you do this with a baby whose eye turns and sticks. Before age three months the child's eye probably won't turn in the direction of a tickle, but we are investing in later habits and

Favouring the phoria with ducky

after three months your cooing and tickling will begin to induce attention and eye movement in the desired direction. The next song will help.

Directional Tromboning

Tromboning is the simple action of moving an interesting object near and far, close to the eye and away. It induces accommodation activity in the lens and activates extrinsic muscles. Use Tromboning to coax, entice or seduce a reluctant eye in the direction you'd like it to go. Anything can be tromboned: a favourite doll, a master of the universe, a plastic dinosaur, a flashy ring, a pink petunia, a piece of toast. A deck of playing cards could be used, or card games from toy stores such as Rummy or Old Maid.

Where Is That Tickle?

Words and Music by Donald Woodward

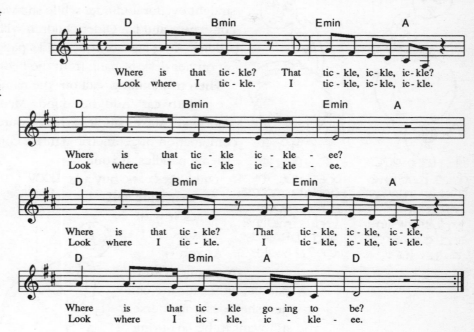

Where is that tic - kle? That tic - kle, ic - kle, ic - kle?
Look where I tic - kle. I tic - kle, ic - kle, ic - kle.

Where is that tic - kle ic - kle - ee?
Look where I tic - kle ic - kle - ee.

Where is that tic - kle? That tic - kle, ic - kle, ic - kle,
Look where I tic - kle. I tic - kle, ic - kle, ic - kle.

Where is that tic - kle go - ing to be?
Look where I tic - kle, ic - kle - ee.

three months to one year

Covering the child's straight or stronger eye with one hand, slowly bring a toy toward and away from her. I discovered that if I sing or murmur while doing this, the baby looks at my mouth instead of the object. When choosing a toy for Directional Tromboning: use objects that twinkle or make a noise.

After the child is four months old, make sure the object is mouthable. She will grab it for spatial exploration with her tongue.

two to ten+ years

Make your own paddles: A paddle is cut out of stiff cardboard in a shape that is easy to hold onto while moving it to and from the eye.

For example, let us make an animal sticker paddle. Cut your piece of cardboard in the shape shown. Then cover it with animal stickers or cut out animals from magazines. I suggest both parent and child

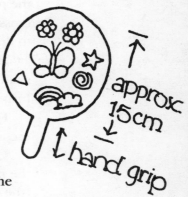

approx 15cm

hand grip

A Tromboning paddle

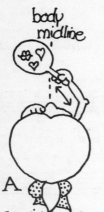

body
midline

A

If right eye
goes out, the
paddle moves
across your
body's midline
and outwards
to the left

B

If left eye
goes out, the
paddle moves
across your
body's midline
and outwards
to the right

have a paddle. Tromboning keeps parents from needing ever reading glasses. Younger children can sit on your lap. Your child may be contented for you to cover her straight eye for a minute while she watches her paddle come near and far. Older children will hold their own paddles. After age six your child's paddle collection can sit on her desk or hang from the bedpost.

When tromboning, call out the name of an animal - e.g. 'kitty cat'. Add the sound. 'Meow'; 'Cow. Mooooo'. Make paddles with coloured circles or combination of geometric figures; construct favourite theme paddles. If your child likes cars, buy a car magazine and attack it with scissors.

As you trombone with the paddle, either for the child or when she does it for herself, you still want to be favouring the phoria each time.

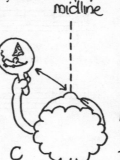
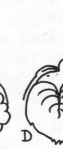

body midline

body midline

C

D

If left eye goes in, the paddle moves away from your body's midline to the left

If right eye goes in, the paddle moves away from your body's midline toward the right

For an eye that drifts outward, cover the other eye and hold the paddle in front of you. Trombone the paddle in and out crossing the midline of your body to draw the eye toward your nose (figures A and B).

Hum, croon, drone, tone, tiddle a ditty as you trombone. This switches on the right side of the brain. The paddle pictures will in turn attract the turning eye back on stage.

For an eye that pulls too far inward, the moving paddle is used to escort the eye in an outward direction (figures C and D).

Covering the opposite eye with the palm of the hand, trombone the paddle from the nose outward, away from the midline of your (the child's) body.

'Photographing' the light

Instructions in this section are addressed to the adult who will then guide the child.

188

six to ten+ years

You and your child should stand with your backs to a light source such as a standing lamp. Turn the lamp so the bulb is visible. Make sure the lamp is incandescent. Never use a suntanning bulb. The sun could be used as a light source also, in the morning or late afternoon, as you will be moving across it only briefly.

Cover the straight eye with the palm of your hand. Both eyes remain open. Keeping your feet in the same spot, do a swing with your whole body around to the light source. Circle the light once then close both eyes and let your body swing back to its original position. After doing this a few times, you will notice that the after-image of the light bulb on your eyelid has moved in the direction you want your turned eye to go. Adults, please experiment with this until you get it right yourself, then teach it to your child.

Phoria ball games

Every child loves a ball. Her first one may be a soft, chewy type. Then come the ones that jingle as they roll. The bouncy, big ones are hot stuff to throw for toddlers. Then you start to play catch. Please make dropping the ball part of the game. No Little League competition here. Collect balls and keep them in a box or basket for phoria play at first and later to play with while Patching.

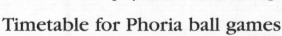

Timetable for Phoria ball games

four months to one+ years

Hide a ball and have it emerge from a surprising place.

Swing a foam ball decorated wildly with glitz and glitter on an elastic string.

one to five+ years

Roll the ball all over your body while laughing and massaging.

Take all the round fruit out of a fruit bowl and roll it to your child.

Bounce a ball on the ground on the side favouring the phoria.

Call your child's name and send the ball to her.

five to ten+ years

Play soccer with your child; as goal-keep always kick the ball to the side favouring the phoria.

Play table tennis and hit the ball to the side that favours the phoria.

Put a foam ball in paint and roll it on paper.

Play with glass marbles, placing the holes or goals on the side favouring the Phoria.

Play catch with a ball. Pretend it is a hot potato.

Buy coloured beach balls to throw on the side Favouring the Phoria. Call out the colours.

Throw a ball against a wall, turn around before it comes down to the side where the turned eye has to look first.

Always talk to each other favouring the phoria.

Who's That In The Mirror?

four months to two years

While your child is still light enough, hold her in front of you; both facing the same way. Stand with your backs to a mirror. Swivel your bodies toward the mirror, keeping your feet facing forward. Exclaim and crow when you see your reflections. 'Who's that in the mirror?' 'Why, it's Joanie!' If you are turning in the correct direction for favouring the phoria, Joanie's inward turning eye will be stimulated to move outward by the

The Mirror Swing

Words and Melody by Helen M. Kennedy

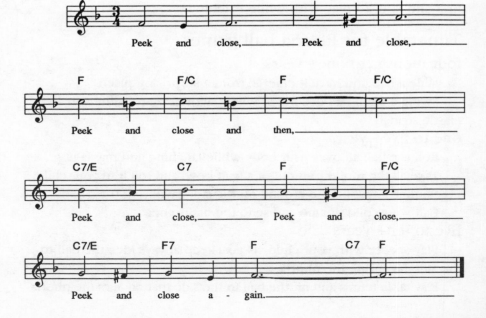

Help Your Child to Perfect Eyesight

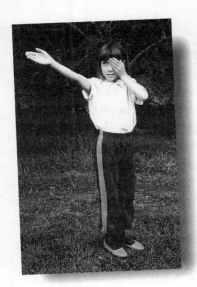

Felicity shows you how to do the Windmill Swing for a right eye that goes in

happy sight of herself. If Joanie's eye is turning outward, you will have to swing across your midline so the turned eye is coaxed toward her nose. Sing this song (page 190).

The Windmill Swing

If your right eye is going inward, stand erect with your feet planted on the ground. Cover your left eye with your left hand. Pretend you right arm is a windmill. Swing it up and back, round and round. Follow your swinging hand with your right eye. In your hand you might like to hold an imaginary owl who has come to have a ride on the windmill.

If your left eye wanders inward, cover your right eye with your right hand. Pretend your left arm is a windmill. Swing it up and back, round and round. Follow your swinging hand with your left eye. Perhaps a giant orange and black monarch butterfly would like to take a ride on your finger tip.

The Windmill Song was written by Helen Kennedy. When she passed away in Los Angeles her family gifted all her Corbett teaching materials to me. Helen had taught hundreds of children to see clearly with straight eyes.

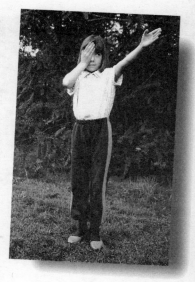

This is the movement if your left eye goes in

The Windmill Swing

Words and Melody by Helen M. Kennedy

Dedicated with love and admiration to Margaret D. Corbett

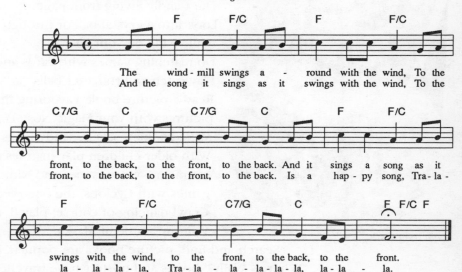

The wind-mill swings a-round with the wind, To the
And the song it sings as it swings with the wind, To the

front, to the back, to the front, to the back. And it
front, to the back, to the front, to the back. Is a

sings a song as it
hap-py song, Tra-la-

swings with the wind, to the front, to the back, to the front.
la - la-la-la, Tra-la - la - la-la-la, la-la - la.

Pirate Patching

Patching the straight eye gives the turning eye a chance to come on stage by itself for a time. The visual brain that belongs to the unpatched eye will be stimulated. Obtain your eye patches from chemists, drug stores or bright coloured ones by mail order from us.

Medical patching often is not effective because the child is totally miserable. This memory lingers in the nervous system. The joy of interacting with others, music and games should be connected with patching, as opposed to the trauma, poison and pain of other methods. Misery switches off the right brain and keeps it off. This inhibits brain integration, a prerequisite for fused eyes.

The brain needs an invitation to help eye muscles relax and vibrate, give and take. Coercion is 99 percent ineffective and counter-productive in any learning process. A new language is best learned while listening to Mozart, switching on both sides of the brain. A new visual habit is best instilled with right-brain levity.

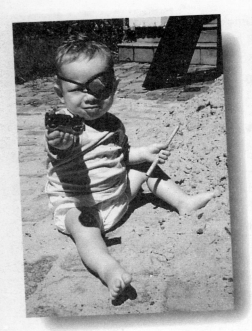

Aerro the pirate

Games to play when pirating

Cross-Crawl dancing

Bird Swing

Near-Far Swing

Circle and count

The Candle Swing from page

Look into a crystal ball or through a quartz crystal while lying on your back

Do matching games with cards and pictures

Play catch and run after balls

Read a picture book. Favouring the phoria, edge the pictures with your Magic Nose Pencil

Make cookies, salads, sandwiches - Pirate food

With older children play marbles or tiddly winks, slot car racing, video games and Nintendo. Do role playing games with Cyclops, the one-eyed monster. Do Cross-Crawl dancing of course; play 'I spy' and 'I went to visit my auntie in Alaska.'

'Search and find' picture books are popular. Martin Handford's 'Where's Wally?' books and posters have travelled around the globe.

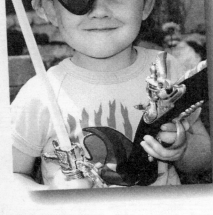

Dale the pirate

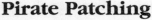 Help Your Child to Perfect Eyesight

'Where's Wendy?' designed by Anthony Tallarico is a less violent version of a finding game. An exciting picture riddle book with photographic realism is 'I Spy, a Book of Picture Riddles' by Walter Wick and Jean Marzollo. For the older members of this age group, I recommend 'For Eagle Eyes Only' and 'Ultimaze' by Rolf Heinmann.

Make this song a family heirloom.

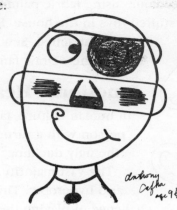

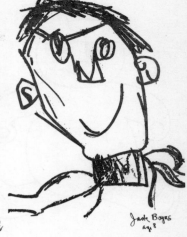

Heave ho, me Hearties!

"Heave Ho! Me Hearties!"

With a Swing   Words and Music by Michael Woodward (Aged 8)

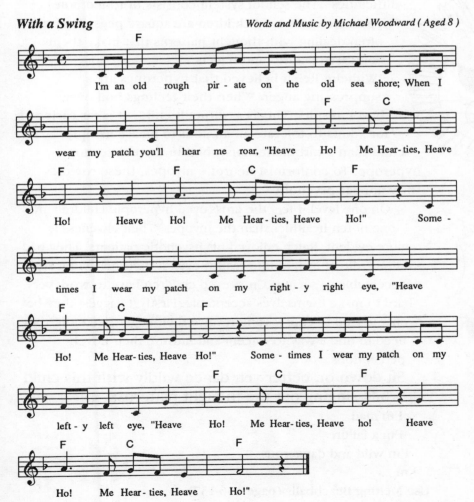

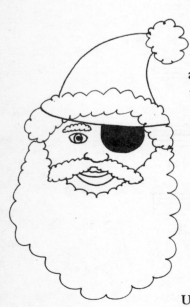

Decorate your eye patches. Do them up in football team colours using fabric paints. Take a scarf and patch all the stuffed toys in the house. Have a collection of hats with patches attached. Sew sequins, ribbons, fabric patches to eye patches. Draw family patching portraits.

Emotional Healing for strabismus

In human culture, fairy-tales and schoolyards, any person with a turned eye is the wicked stepsister, the ugly duckling.

The vast majority of children with turned eyes are also hyperopic. This group of people have the challenge of playing the misfits in the school system. They are most often designated as the ones with 'learning difficulties'. The school system consists of round holes. Hyperopic cross-eyed children are square pegs. They are often dealing with thought patterns that make them outcasts, failures and rejects.

Wilhelm Reich believed that hyperopes are suppressing anger. When their feelings boil over, havoc results. This is a 'difficult child.' It is far easier for adults to tolerate an anxious-to-please myopic child than a turbulent, noisy, bull in the china shop hyperope. To conformist neurotic myopes, these rowdies may appear psychotic

On one level, I feel the cross-eyed hyperopic children are one notch healthier than the myopes. Their aliveness is more evident. Reich enjoyed his psychotic patients. They had a unique, direct insight into reality, even if their behaviour was unacceptable to society. Cross-eyed children have to work very hard to make themselves acceptable. Firstly, I suggest they be encouraged to express and resolve their anger. Secondly, they need to find a way to esteem and nurture their novel perceptions.

Sit down or, better yet, dance wildly with this child while singing out the thought patterns:

I'm mad

I'm a failure

I'm wild and dangerous

I'm....

Use Melting Beachballs (page 136-137).

Help Your Child to Perfect Eyesight

Some word patterns I've heard from cross-eyed children

I'm ugly	I'm beautiful
I'm crooked	I'm straight
I don't fit in here	This is my place

The nasty step-sister with a cast in her eye in fairy-tales is an archetype representing the ugly side of ourselves that we all want to reject. Strabismic children, consciously or unconsciously, have the special task of transmuting this rejected side of humanity. This is true, even if yours is the cutest cross-eyed child in the world. It is a unique opportunity for us all to deal with the part of us that we condemn. Loving ourselves when we are ugly <u>and</u> when we are beautiful is the key.

Using the Beachballs, place 'I'm ugly' in one hand. Give your Beachball a colour. Make it huge. Yell 'I'm ugly' to the sky or whisper it to the Easter bunny. Express it, until you are satisfied with the size, weight and colour of your 'I'm ugly' beachball.

Then ask, 'What is the opposite of ugly?' Some children may have a different expression. If it is 'I'm cute,' put 'I'm cute,' or 'I'm handsome' in the opposite hand. Expand the phrase with sound and colour into a Beachball that somehow equals the first Beachball. When this occurs smoosh the two Beachballs together with passion, with a sound - with an explosion or implosion. Bring your smooshed Beachballs to your heart and release them.

Have a good time with this song.

The Cross-Eyed Monster

Music - Traditional
Words by Janet Goodrich

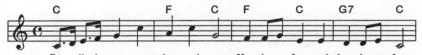

I'm a lit-tle mon-ster, short and stout. Here is my fang and here is my clout.

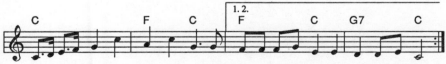

I'm a lit-tle mon-ster, cross-eyed too, and When I turn my eyes in, you turn to glue.
When I turn my eyes in, I'm scar-ing you.

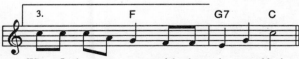

When I keep my eyes straight the sky turns blue!

Timetable for strabismus

birth to one year

Occasionally hold your hand over the straight eye - only for as long as she will tolerate it. Use directional tromboning, Who's That in the Mirror?, songs and finger plays.

one to five+ years

From the age of imitation (ten to 24 months) onward, patching should be a social affair. Other family members can use patches while games are played. As soon as the patch is bothersome it comes off or sits on the top of the head. Using this approach, children have carried patches to their parents saying, 'Let's sing Heave Ho!' and 'Aren't you going to use your patch?'

five+ years

Use Directional tromboning, 'Photographing' the light, and the Windmill Swing.

Heading for fusion

You must decide when your child is ready to play the fusion games in the next chapter. You don't want to rush matters, but it may occur faster than you think.

All the directional games in this chapter are preparation for binocular vision. Follow your intuition. Most likely you and your child will be shifting back and forth between directional games, Patching and fusion activities.

Chapter Seventeen

Fusion

What is fusion?

Fusion is binocular, or two-eyed vision. It occurs when the messages from both eyes are used together by the visual brain. Only the images from the macula lutea are fused. Even though you don't notice, all contours and shapes peripheral to your small area of central fused vision are double. Hold the tip of your finger about 15 cm (six inches) in front of your nose. Centre your attention on your fingertip. Notice that all the other objects in the room, all the items you're not looking at, are double. They will be double unless you are using the message from only one of your eyes.

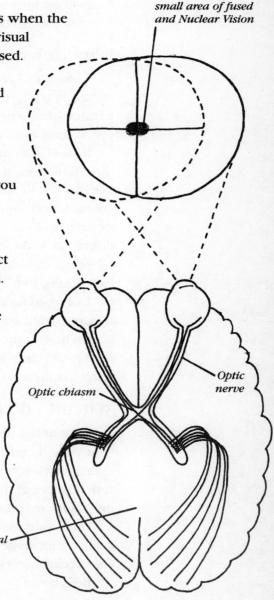

Macula lutea, the small area of fused and Nuclear Vision

The physical side of fusion

This illustration shows how optic nerves connect eyeballs to the visual cortex in the back of the head.

Notice that the optic nerves meet at the optic chiasm. Here they shake hands and trade some nerve fibres, but only those from one side of their respective visual fields. Part of the visual field from the right eye leads to the left side of the visual cortex; and part of the visual field from the left eye leads to the right side of the visual cortex. The result? The left visual cortex gets handed the messages from the right side of the visual field from both your left and your right eye, and vice versa. Are you confused? It's an intriguing design. It works just fine until stress or trauma interferes.

Optic chiasm

Optic nerve

Reasons for not fusing

Accident or disease can destroy fusion ability. If the eyes are physically *Primary visual cortex where fusion takes place* healthy, but there is a turned eye, the image from a turning eye may be put on hold by the brain. This was explained in the previous chapter on strabismus.

Since fusion is mainly directed from the brain a restriction or illness that interferes with normal brain development could sabotage fusion. Another reason could be a large difference in the refractive error of each eye.

There is an emotional and mental side to fusion. The process of regaining fusion brings up powerful feelings. These feelings and their companion memories may be a primary cause of continued resistance to fusion.

Why is fusion important?

Unbalanced fusion leads to eyestrain and fatigue. Physical energy is used in trying to force a misaligned eye to stay in line with its partner. Even when the brain decides to suppress the image from one eye, it must burn energy to do so (page 179).

Balanced binocular vision brings with it distinct advantages. Full three-dimensional perception comes from blending together the macular lutea ('nuclear') images from each eye, producing rich colour vision and full depth perception. If there are refractive error differences in the eyes, strong fusion helps to neutralise the discrepancy. Persons with -5 diopters in one eye and -1 diopter in the other may benefit tremendously from fusion games. With few exceptions, two eyes see better together than each eye separately.

Disturbed fusion and the three common refractive errors - myopia, hyperopia and astigmatism - are all the result of an imbalance somewhere in the child's being. Occasionally take all children through the four levels of fusion as a helpful adjunct to their programmes for refractive error; even when fusion is not the main problem.

When to do fusion games

Most of the fusion games in this chapter require special time with your child. I consider them suitable for ages five and up. At least once a week you could say, 'Let's meet Thursday evening to play fusion games at the kitchen table.' If you can get in a second session on Sunday morning that will be even better.

Once your child gets to the stage where he is familiar with fusion games, encourage him to teach them to other children. Young people are excellent teachers. Knowledge passed on solidifies in the giver.

Before you do fusion games together, warm up with Cross-Crawl dancing and Palming. Use Emotional Healing for fusion as needed. Adults have burst into tears on seeing with fusion for the first time in a vision class. Other students became cranky when they didn't get the Gate described below. Expect sparks and carry tissues.

When doing fusion games it is important to return continually to relaxation, Yawning, and Cross-Crawl. Use lots of praise and recognition of baby steps in healing fusion. If your child sees the Gate for half a second, pause for jubilation. That may even be enough success for one session.

Do not allow your disapproval of turned eyes to flavour the game. Keep yourself free of fairy-tale prejudices the best you can. After all that - let's get to some action!

Fusion Level One: the Gate

Place your finger about 15 cm (six inches) directly in front of your nose. Edge something in **the distance beyond your finger** with your Magic Nose Pencil.

You may notice that your finger appears doubled and blurred. We call this phenomenon 'the Gate'. It comes when you have fusion, when you are using the images from both eyes.

If you do not have the Gate, you might be looking directly at your finger. Please send your attention into the distance. If your gate still doesn't appear, your visual brain may have turned off the image from one of your eyes.

Sometimes it takes a while for the second image to click in, so be patient with this if it doesn't occur right away.

If the second finger doesn't appear at all, see what happens with the Fantastic Fusion Fixer (FFF).

Cut a piece of stiff cardboard about 10 cm (4 inches) wide and 15 cm (6 inches) long. The card should have complimentary colors on either side for high contrast: bright red with the other side green, one side blue and the other orange, or yellow and purple. Pasting together two pieces of different coloured construction paper will do. You could also colour or paint some white paper.

Glue to one side of the card a picture of a brilliant flower or animal. Make sure the image contrasts highly with the background

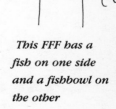

This FFF has a fish on one side and a fishbowl on the other

colour on that side of the card. Put a bee on the other side.

Hold the card in front of your nose snug enough to your face so that your right eye sees only the right side of the card and your left eye sees only the left side of the card.

While holding the FFF card in front of your nose, cover your right eye with a hand or another card. Notice, absorb and memorise the side of the card you see with this eye. Alternately: cover your left eye with your hand or another card. Notice, absorb and memorise the side of the card you see with this eye.

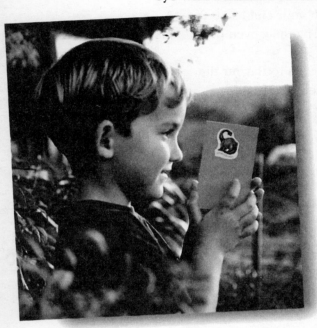

Will is looking at a flower in the distance through his FFF.

Close both eyes. With your eyes closed remember and visualise the left eye's side of the card to the right of your nose. Visualise the right eye's side of the card to the left of your nose. Now **imagine the two sides of the card at the same time.** I agree it's tricky. The cards switch sides because your optic nerves trade fibres, as mentioned above.

Open both eyes. Say, 'Hurrah!' if both sides of the card, the bee and the flower, appear at the same time, even for a split second. Repeat this activity at other times until you have a solid, lasting experience of binocular vision.

Straight eyes but no fusion?

It is possible to have both eyes straight, with no large difference in the refractive error of the two eyes, but still not have fusion. The message from one eye is being used, the other message is playing second fiddle. In this case Patching is helpful to encourage the eye that is not being fully utilised to catch up.

Deciding which eye to patch

When there is a turning eye, it is easy to determine. The patch goes on the straight eye. In the case where it is not so obvious, use the Fantastic Fusion Fixer to discover which eye is not being used. Switch the card around several times, letting each eye have a chance to view the flower. If the flower consistently **disappears when it's on the right side** of your nose then your brain may be turning off the messages from your right eye. Therefore you would **patch your left eye.**

If the flower consistently **disappears on the left side** of your

👁 Help Your Child to Perfect Eyesight

nose then your brain may be turning off the messages from your left eye. Therefore you would **patch your right eye.**

Cover up the 'good eye' and play some movement vision games for a while. If you do put on an eye patch fusion games won't work; because you will only get fusion if you have two uncovered functioning eyes. After Patching for a while, return to fusion games and see what happens.

Fusion Level Two: the Bug and Bead Game

Take a piece of string about two metres (six ft) long. Two people each hold one end of the string or tie one end to a convenient structure. You should end up sitting about one metre (three ft) away from where the string is fastened to person, chair or railing. Wind your end of the string around your forefinger and hold it 15 cm (six in) in front of your chin. Don't hold the string too tightly to your chin. You want to be able to move your head around easily.

Place a brightly coloured bead on your string. If two people are holding the string each will have their own bead. If you can't find a bead in your house, use a paper clip, a small hair band, a piece of thick yarn or a diamond ring. Slide the bead outward until it is sitting 25cm (10 inches) from your hand.

Now that you are all set with your string and bead, close your eyes and pretend you have a pet bug flying around in the room. It could be a bee, a butterfly, a pterodactyl, a space ship or whatever you like. Your bug or UFO love aerial acrobatics. It performs loop-de-loops and triple somersaults with the greatest of ease. You follow your bug with your nose of course. (This can be done first with a real object, a toy for example, until we have the idea, then use your imagination.)

After your bug has finished showing off, it will come in for a landing exactly on your bead.

Blink your eyes open and circle the bug on your bead with your nose. What do you notice? Do you have one string or two? Has the string you are holding with one hand magically made itself into two strings? If it has, then you are experiencing fusion - which can now be refined with the next question.

Are the two strings meeting and making an 'X' somewhere near your bead with the bug on it?

Case 1 If your 'X' crosses within 2.5cm (one inch) of your bead your mind and your eye muscles are working together.

Congratulations. Grasp the bead with your free hand and give your bug a ride near and far on the string. Breathe and Yawn. This near-far movement with the bead combines both fusion and accommodation. Excellent for reading stamina and a career in computers. Repeat this game only occasionally.

Case 2 If your bead is crossing more than five cm (two inches) **in front of** your bug, put your string down and Trombone out and to the side, favouring the Phoria, for three minutes. Time's up? Stop Tromboning, pick up your string and see if your X is now crossing closer to your bead. Yes, congratulations. If you don't know already what Tromboning is from Chapter 16, here it is:

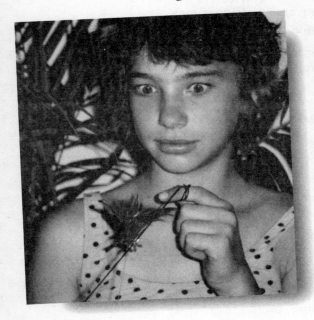

Fuchsia's bug landed on her bead. So did both her eyes.

Tromboning outward for esophoria

Make yourself a paddle of stiff cardboard. Put some brightly coloured stickers or cutouts on the paddle to attract the eye. Because eyes are always attracted to motion and colour, we move the paddle like the slide on a trombone to coax a turned or wandering eye in the direction we want it to go. With Tromboning, overtight muscles relax. (See instructions on page 187.)

For eyes that tend to pull too far inward, the paddle is used to escort the eye in an outward direction. Covering the opposite eye with the palm of the hand, trombone the paddle from your nose outward, away from the centre/mid-line of your body. Humming and crooning will help to stimulate the visual system while easing the eye outward. Change eyes and do the same movement. Do each eye for about three minutes. (See illustration on page 188, Figures C and D.)

The Widening River

The 'Widening River' visualisation is helpful for eyes that are over-converging. These eyes are called esophoric. Esophoria does not have to be so severe as to be labelled strabismus. It is, however, a subtle tendency which can result in brain and eye fatigue.

Put the string and bead away for a while. Palm your eyes and tell a story where you imagine you are standing at the source of a river. The river widens as it flows away in front of you. Trace the side of the river extending out to the right and then the side extending to the left. Fill out your visualisation of the river with fish, turtles and

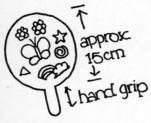

approx 15cm

hand grip

A Tromboning paddle

Help Your Child to Perfect Eyesight

charming mermaids. Two mermaids swim away
from you. They get farther away from one
another as they swim into the distance. They
find their sitting rocks on the horizon and wave at
you. After palming go back to the Bug and Bead.

Case 3 If your 'X' crosses <u>beyond</u> your bead or
you have two parallel lines, then it's time to stop and
do some Tromboning inward for three minutes. Then
return to the bead and string to see if your 'X' has moved
closer to your bead.

Tromboning inward for exophoria

For eyes that tends to drift outward, cover one eye and
hold the paddle in front of you. Trombone the paddle in and out,
crossing the mid-line of your body, noticing the pictures getting
larger and smaller. Hum with the in-and-out rhythm of your paddle.
Humming sounds vibrate skull bones and activate your right-brain.
The paddle attracts and coaxes the eye inward. Do the same action
with your other eye.

Do Tromboning for about three minutes.
(See illustrations on page 188, figures A and B.)

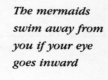

*The mermaids
swim away from
you if your eye
goes inward*

The Precious Shell

Visualising the Precious Shell will help
loosen eye muscles and tell your brain it's OK to
point both your eyes toward the bead at the same
time. Put the string and bead aside for a moment.
Palm your eyes and imagine you are at the seashore.
You stand at the edge of the water looking out toward the
ocean. In the distance on your right is a mermaid sitting on
a rock. Her twin sister is sitting on a rock in the distance to
your left. When you whistle, they both jump into the water and
swim toward you as fast as they can. They are converging on you.
Smiling, their hair dripping seaweed, they each hand you half a
seashell. You must put the two halves of the seashell together
right in front of your eyes.

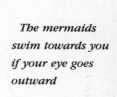

*The mermaids
swim towards you
if your eye goes
outward*

Once your seashell is together, put it in your pocket. Bring
your palms away from your face, blink your eyes open and return to
your string. Is your 'X' now closer to your bead? Congratulations.

If at any time you find you have stiffened up your shoulders, or if
you're turning blue from holding your breath, please take a break.
Yawn like a lion. Do Cross-Crawl dancing before returning to the
Bug on the Bead.

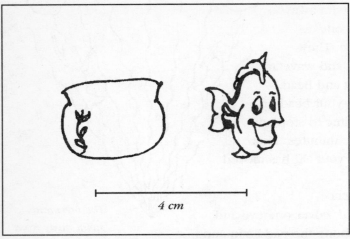

4 cm

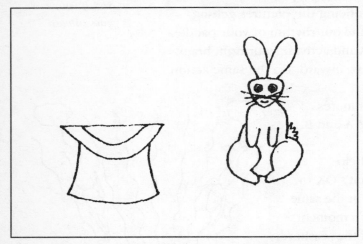

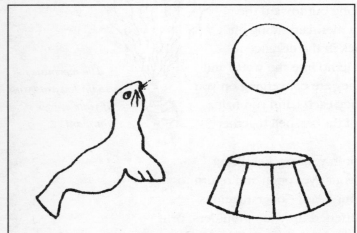

Fusion cards by NVI teacher Shirley Beasley

Note to adults

When playing the Bug and Bead game with a younger child, please do not ask him if he has an 'X'. Phrase the question differently. Ask him what he sees as he holds the string and circles the bug. Once you have a response you can go from there: 'How many strings do you have?' and 'Show me with your free hand where the strings go.'

If he sees two strings (which may or may not cross) you can ask, 'Do the two strings meets anywhere?' and 'Where do they cross?'.

Fusion Level Three: Fish in a Bowl

More fusion fun can be had by children who are already seeing the Gate at least part of the time if they use fusion cards they have made themselves. Using these cards will help their visual brain get more into the fusion habit.

On a plain piece of paper or card just the right size to hold in your hand, draw a fishbowl on one side, and on the other side, a fish. Draw the pictures 4 cm (1.5 in) apart because that is the easiest distance for the visual system to overlap two images when the card is held 25 cm (10 in) in front of your nose.

At first you may get four images, two fish and two fishbowls. Realise that it may take a few moments for the fish to overlap with the fishbowl. Breathe, smile and move the card slowly near and far until you hear a splash.

👁 Help Your Child to Perfect Eyesight

The possibilities for fusion card creations are infinite. Make a deck of cards with sport, cooking or musical themes. Let yourselves brainstorm ideas. In brainstorming every idea is accepted, so stir up as many ideas as possible - the wilder the better.

Fusion Level Four: Magic Eyes

When children have a lot of reading and desk work to do or are sitting at computers, their visual system need *fusional reserve*. This means their brain and eye muscle co-ordination has such a strong foundation that even hours of reading (with the Great White Glow) will not make their eyes tired or strained.

The popular 'Magic Eye' books and posters are based on this principle. A child who does not have solid fusion abilities will be left out in the cold when others are exclaiming over the 3-D images that are emerging from the garbled computer-generated graphics.

But once he has developed the Gate and progressed through fusion levels two and three, he should (with relaxation and gentle scanning with his Nose Feather) be able to satisfy his heart.

Magic Eye N.E.
Thing enterprises

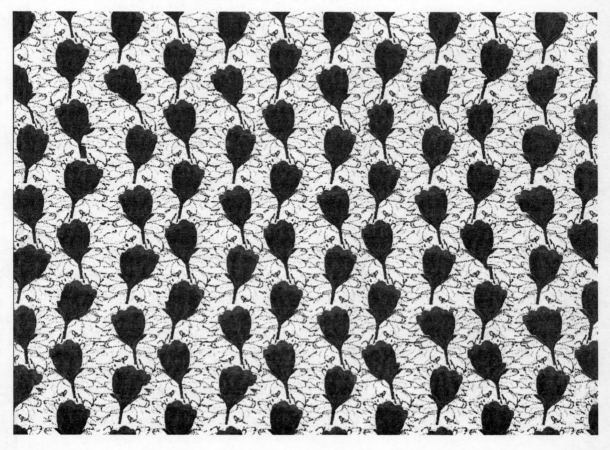

Angel Haloes

Once your child has achieved Fusion Level One - the Gate - you can make him an Angel Halo. There are several ways to make a Halo. You could use pipe-cleaners or soft clothesline wire. But

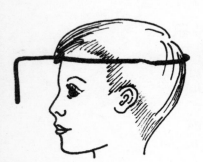

Two kinds of haloes

please do not put the metal circle all the way around the head, as you would be closing off the governing meridian, causing mental scramble and discomfort. We use a rubber band to close the front of a metal Halo that encircles the head.

An alternative is to make a hole in the beak of a baseball cap and push a straight stick through the hole. Children can wear the Halo when reading or doing any other activity. It is especially good for hyperopic children to build fusional reserve.

The vertical part of the Halo should sit at a distance from the child's eyes where the two sides of the gate fall into the margin of the page. Use the Halo while doing the Bird Swing to multiply saccadic movement.

Alternating vision

Alternating strabismus or squint occurs when the child looks at you with the right eye, sending the left eye off to the woods, then looks at you with the left eye, sending the right eye off for a swim. Alternating vision is trainable. With loving persistence you have a good chance of inviting errant eyes back to the same party. Patching will not help in this case. But fusion games with lots of body feeling, excitement and enthusiasm will call in his two eyes to land on your face at the same time.

The following fusion games are based on the irresistible power of imagination and body awareness, the kind we get from swinging on a swing, or dancing. Touching hands and eyes will feed back into the visual brain what it is like to use the messages from both eyes simultaneously.

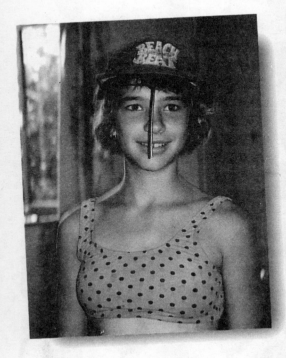

Fuchsia is using a wire Halo under her baseball cap

👁 Help Your Child to Perfect Eyesight

The butterfly mask

Materials needed:

Paper, crayons, Scotch tape, rubber bands or string to fasten the mask on his head.

The illustration shown is an example. Your child could make his own mask. Perhaps he prefers the face of a lion or a Tyrannosaurus Rex.

Cut two eye holes for the mask, making sure they are right in front of the child's eyes. Ask him to find you with his right eye, while holding his right hand in yours. Ask him to find you with his left eye, holding his left hand in yours. Do this several times until you are fairly sure he is aware of which eye he is using. Bring both his hands together saying, 'Find me with both eyes at once.' Give a jubilant AHAH, whether he succeeds or not.

How many times you might be able to repeat this game I don't know. I do know that any kind of change takes love and patience. Be assured that your child's brain will be mulling over the possibilities. Do this game for three minutes each time - longer if he wants to.

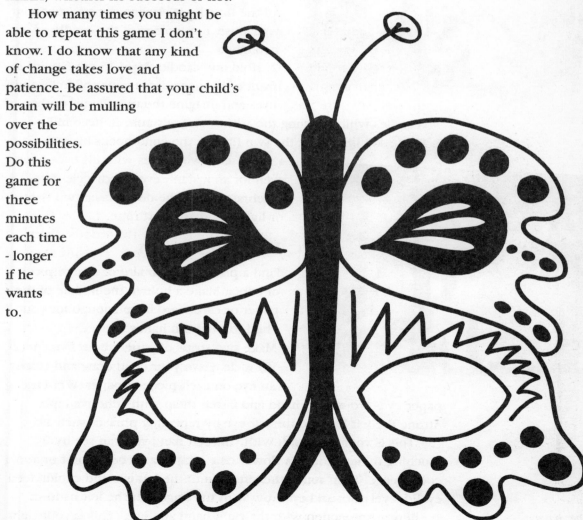

Candles in the Dark

Materials needed:

Two candles, a coloured sticker to put on your nose, a darkened room. Note: Two penlights would work equally well.

1. In your darkened room hold two lit candles about 15 cm (six in) in front of your child and about 5 cm (two in) apart. Put a sticker or a coloured mark on the end of your nose. Tell the child, 'This is what you will see when you are fusing'.

Now hold one candle in front of him and say, 'This one light will magically turn into two candles like this.' (Again hold up the two candles about five cm (two in) apart. All the time he is circling the sticker on your nose, not looking at the candle or penlight.)

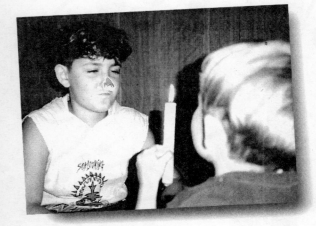

2. Hold one candle about 15 cm (six in) in front of his nose: Have your child close his eyes and imagine the two flames of the candles whilst circling the sticker on your nose in his mind.

3. While still imagining the two flames, the child opens his eyes.

4. If he sees two flames with his eyes open even for an instant, everybody celebrate. Celebrate even if he doesn't see two flames or lights. Perhaps next time.

Feeling Fusion

Find a piece of cardboard or a large piece of paper. Make a hole in the middle of the paper or cardboard large enough for your child to put both hands in.

Make two strips of paper about five cm (2 in) wide. Have your child draw and colour an eye on each piece of paper. Wrap the paper eyes around his hand and fasten them with adhesive tape. Attune the left hand to the left eye by repeating phrases such as:

'This is your left hand. With your left hand you can see by touching things.' Touch a flower or a rock or a piece of toast or a cool breeze. Then touch the left hand to the left eye and explore eyelid, eyelashes and eyebrow with the fingers of the left hand.

Repeat this action with the right hand and eye: 'This is your right

👁 Help Your Child to Perfect Eyesight

hand. With your right hand you can see by touching things. Touch a piece of wood, my nose, the water in this glass.' Then repeat these rhymes and take appropriate action.

My right eye is a rabbit,   **or**   My right eye is an aeroplane,
My left eye is a hare.   My left eye is one too.
When they see their hole -   When they see Fusion Bay -
They both jump right in there.   They fly into the blue!

Use the hands again to get the feeling of fusion deep, deep into the body and mind. In your left hand is a lake. Close your eyes and imagine the lake. In your right hand is a moon. The moon and the lake splash together. In your left hand is a red banana pie. In your right hand is a blue banana pie. Squish the two pies together. What do you get?

Your two hands are lanterns glowing fiercely outdoors on a dark windy night. Take a big breath and bring the two glowing lamps together. What do you get?

If your child is old enough, you could experiment with bringing together the flames of two candles. First for real, then in the imagination. Always do the motions with hands and arms even when imagining. The kinesthetic movement of the body feeds the feeling of fusion into the brain.

After tuning up body and brain for fusion, take the child with alternating vision back to level one - the Gate. See what happens.

If you and your child dream up new ideas and games for finding fusion, please send them to me. Your ideas will be shared with other families.

Emotional Healing for fusion

The essence of fusion is joining together and cooperation. The right eye and right side of the body directed through the left-brain represents the male aspect and father. Mother and the feminine is represented by the left eye, left side of the body and the right brain. Male and female union within oneself is as vulnerable to disruption as getting married in America. One out of three unions end in divorce.

Cameron Dawson finds that 30 percent of his patients have fusion problems ranging from hardly noticeable to grossly strabismic.

Statements to play with

I see with one eye	I see with both eyes
I am cock-eyed	My eyes are balanced

There is a silent internal argument going on. When this conflict is made audible it sounds something like this:

I want to be separate	I want to join together
I must be single	I am everything
I will be destroyed by others	Others uplift me
I must look out for myself	I am safe

Use Melting Beachballs to clarify and dissolve blocked feelings. Not every child will have the same thought patterns. Start out simply by placing the fact in your left hand: 'I see with one eye.' Make it into an energy ball with colour, size and weight. Repeat the words out loud with enthusiasm, making your Beachball grow in size and effect until the rocks and oceans notice it. Now ask the question: 'Can you love yourself even when you see with one eye?' If the answer is yes, then ask for the opposite of seeing with one eye. Put that response in a huge Beachball in your right hand: 'I see with both eyes together at the same time.' Build up this statement with colour and impact. When your two balls balance each other and you are satisfied with your expressions, implode your two balls together right in front of you. Bring your hands to your heart and go on with your life.

Timetable for fusion

birth to eight months

During this homolateral phase it's too early for fusion games. Do swinging and directional games if your baby has a turned eye.

eight months to one year

This is the building and solidifying phase for fusion. In general, sit back and watch the baby crawl in his own time. If your child needs help, you can do manual Cross-Crawling. You grasp his right hand and bring it to his left foot and vice versa. Do this not more than ten times in a session.

two to four years

Continue with directional Tromboning and Swings (if needed) from Chapter 16.

four to six years

Experiment with the Gate, using metre or yardsticks, coloured pens and home-made fusion cards.

Help Your Child to Perfect Eyesight

six to 10+ years

Start with the Gate, then go on to Fusion Level Two, the Bug and Bead Game. Take children slowly and patiently through Fusion Levels One to Four. Return frequently to easy fusion games where kids can be successful. Edge yourselves slowly and delicately toward more advanced levels.

Part Four

Home and school environments

Chapter Eighteen

Sugar and sore eyes

Bodies are made of food

Just as a factory needs raw materials to produce a go-cart or a computer, children need raw materials of a particular kind to produce healthy body parts. Vitamins, minerals and proteins are the necessary ingredients. Every newborn is gifted with an immense ability to recover. Every child comes in with reservoirs of enzymes and minerals. The diet of the mother while pregnant has an effect; and what goes into the child's body in the next years will determine her moods and affect her physical health. If she lives on empty calories, her reservoirs will be depleted, rather than replenished.

It looks as if children can eat anything. They have strong digestions, pink cheeks and bounding energy. Sometimes it takes twelve years of junk food to produce a teenager with poor eyesight, sugar addictions (teenage alcoholism is a major problem in the USA), depression and problems in school.

The person buying the groceries determines the diet patterns of the rest of the family. Starting children out with foods that contain the building blocks for the body is a challenge. Do what you can before and during the high-chair phase. You will have to educate relatives and friends who come offering sweets. This requires daily practice. It will take shopping-bag awareness. It could mean changing what you eat.

A thorough discussion of foods and their relationship to the eye, brain and mind complex would require another book. I had to decide on a key element. White sugar. Why do I pick on white sugar?

Sugar is the ultimate challenge. Having raised three children in a sugar culture, I know the pitfalls and opposing forces. If you can divert (or even blow up) the sugar train, your desire to promote any other healthy dietary habits will be easy. If you as a parent or care-giver to children can produce a child who will buy an apple rather than a candy bar, I salute you. At 15 she may be making salads and steaming vegetables without being asked. Another reason why I have chosen white sugar is that white sugar has been linked to developing myopia.

Sugar blues

The World Health Organization listed processed sugar as one of the five substances to which citizens of industrial nations are addicted. Dare I call processed sugar a drug? My dictionary says a drug is a chemical substance taken for the pleasant effect it produces. I learned, when first giving weekend vision improvement seminars, to ask the organizers to whisk away the coffee and sugar packets.

'Also get rid of these cookies and sweet biscuits!' I didn't quite bellow. All my myopic students were nodding off at three o'clock in the afternoon. When I spoke of sugar highs and sugar lows, a 16 year-old protested, 'I thought sugar gives you energy.' Yes, for a short period, then it opens a trapdoor under your feet. Simple sugar over-stimulates the pancreas. Complex sugars, as found in fruits and vegetables, stay with you longer. The pancreas is related to feelings of apathy: 'I just can't move.' On the second day of the seminar apples and oranges were served.

Excessive sugar in the body is eliminated partially through the eyes. 'Sleep'(the crystalline crust found in your eyes in the morning) is often caused by the sweets you ate yesterday.

This drug is not an outlaw. It's everywhere. In relation to vision problems it is our first and main wrestling partner.

Your child's visual field is plastered with the shape, colour and taste of soft drinks and candy. Chocolate, cheap and exclusive, is the taste that consoles, congratulates and celebrates. Let's take a look at chocolate candy bars in relationship to the visual blur called myopia.

All chocolate contains white sugar and oxalic acid. White sugar in the body sneaks into its mineral storehouse and steals away chromium. What's chromium? It's a trace mineral. Lack of chromium is a factor in the development of myopia.

Oxalic acid slows down the rate at which calcium is absorbed in the body. Calcium is essential for strong teeth and bones. It's the reason why we are told to drink our milk. Yet the calcium in milk is insoluble in the human body. Cow's milk products have had excellent press and advertising. More people are finding out that it is not fit for human consumption. The chocolate milk we were given in our school lunches contained the worst of both worlds. One sign of lack of calcium is increased myopia.

It is an illusion to increase the intake of calcium-bearing foods such as milk and cheese in the hope that your body will take calcium out of these foods and put it in the right places. Calcium works in partnership with magnesium. Some doctors believe that high calcium intake of the wrong kind causes premature aging, pre-menstral tension and osteoporosis. Rather than forcing ice cream, cheese and milk down children, it is advised to increase magnesium. One of the best ways to do this is to cook peasant food for your family. This means foods like whole grain millet, barley and rye. Millet contains eight parts magnesium to one part calcium. Use these grains cooked as breakfast cereals. After soaking grains overnight use them sprouted and mixed with vegies as cold salads.

Sugar hit parade

The child's world is sprinkled with white sugar; cakes, cookies and candy bars. 'Empty calories' they are called, for they have no body-building value. In my dream I entered our local general store. Glitter and sparkle, purple, green, gold dazzled my eyes from the floor to eight feet. Inside the glitzy flat or lumpy parcels were nuggets of sweet browness. Three girls, just losing their baby teeth, stood at the counter with sweaty pocket coins in one hand, their selections in the other. Doing research for this book, I asked them why they were spending their pocket money on candy. A blue-eyed blondy replied, "It's got tattoos in it." The second grinned, "I can win a prize." The third little girl glared at me "I like the taste."

You must cope with advertisements on TV, birthday parties, school parties and festivals. Soft drinks can contain up to 60 percent white sugar. What can you do? Gain some understanding of the chemical and emotional significance of sugar consumption. Then find and use at home and school as many substitution ideas as possible.

Emotionally sugar is the taste of the past. It soothes and pacifies like suckling at the breast. Chocolate stimulates endorphins, which are chemical relaxants and pleasure hormones in the brain. Sugar is a drug that reminds people of past comforts. It is eaten by people yearning for love. Chocolate contains caffeine, a stimulant and toxin. That's a double whammy surrogate adventure story that ends in a crumbling crystal palace. It's a transitory addictive illusion that weakens bodies and minds. One therapy for addictions is to over-do it. Try living only on chocolate for a couple of weeks observing your behaviour and thoughts. Or consider taking in minerals.

Why people want sugar

People who crave sugar are **lacking in minerals**. Refined and processed foods, such as cakes, candies, cookies, cereals, white rice and white bread, have been stripped of vitamins and minerals. Foods grown on soil replenished only with phosphate and nitrogenous fertilizers are lacking in trace minerals.

It's a vicious circle. The child is missing minerals and experiences this lack as a longing for sugar. Sugar enters the blood stream, giving a rise in energy. Children call this a 'sugar hit'. Blood sugar levels rise rapidly triggering an alarm that races through the body crying out 'Too much sugar here. Get rid of it.' The body obeys and blood sugar drops suddenly. Your marvellous vital angel transforms into a tired rag doll or an irritable brat.

The culprit being discussed here is refined white sugar. More complex sugars such as those in fruit and fruit juices do not cause the same highs and lows in blood sugar levels as does white sugar. 'Why does Steve have constant headaches?' his mother asked me after a vision class. I turned around and asked ten year-old Steve, 'How much soda pop are you drinking?' 'Two bottles of Pepsi a day,' he said. When fruit juice was substituted for the sugared carbonated water, Steve's headaches stopped. Vegetables and grains contain complex carbohdyrates (sugar and starch molecules) which take even longer to break down in the body. These are the foods that 'stay with you'.

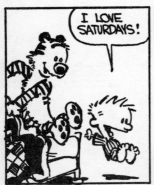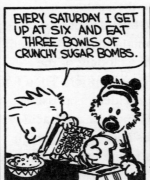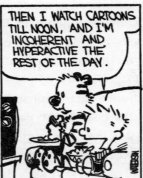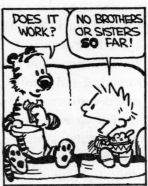

What you can do

Complaining doesn't work. 'You're eating too much candy' can bring out a rebel response.

What works is to eat right yourself — at least during the age of imitation, which is birth to age five. During this time eating habits are established. Baby Aerro was fed mainly vegetables, whole-cooked grains and fruit. On his first birthday the celebrating adults decided to buy a chocolate cake, something Aerro had never seen. A piece

Help Your Child to Perfect Eyesight

was put in his mouth. Everyone laughed at the wry expression on his face. Aerro spurned more cake and crawled over to my plate to gobble up green peas.

Get minerals into your body. Vegetables and whole grains contain minerals. If you live in a region where you suspect the vegetables are grown on depleted soil, then consider buying a mineral supplement. Ask at your health food store, drugstore or chemist for a mineral supplement that would be suitable for both yourself and your child.

Fill your shopping bag with fresh fruit and vegetables rather than squishy things in shiny, coloured wrappers. Yes, our eyes are attracted to glitz, but also to bright oranges and slippery bananas.

Buy unsweetened fruit juices and dilute to a proportion of two parts juice to one part water. Make ice-blocks of this in summer.

Look for recipe books on healthy food for children.

People with hypoglycemia (low blood sugar) are told to eat protein rather than simple sugars. There is lots of protein in nuts and seeds. To restore enzyme activity, soak sunflower seeds, almonds, hazelnuts or peanuts in water overnight or for six hours. Pour the water off and rinse in a sieve. Keep them in the refrigerator if they are not eaten up the first day. They are crunchy, fulfilling, and visually interesting. They start to grow.

For snacks, carry apples, oranges, carrots, celery, rice crackers, nuts, dates, and raisins.

I'd Like To Be

Words and Music by Donald Woodward

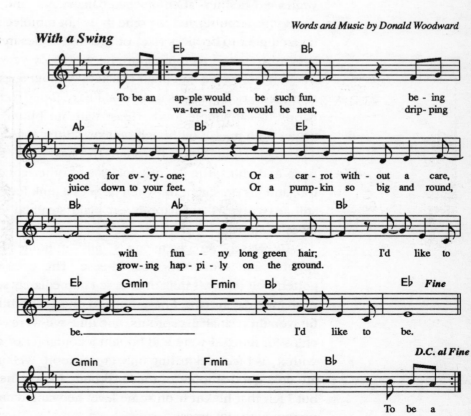

With a Swing

To be an ap-ple would be such fun, be-ing
wa-ter-mel-on would be neat, drip-ping

good for ev-'ry-one; Or a car-rot with-out a care,
juice down to your feet. Or a pump-kin so big and round,

with fun-ny long green hair; I'd like to
grow-ing hap-pi-ly on the ground.

be. I'd like to be.

To be a

Add your own rhymes about fruit and vegetables you like!

As sweeteners use 'real' sugars such as honey (remembering that some people cannot use honey because it is too concentrated), maple syrup, dates, rice and apple syrup.

See if you can get school chocolate sales turned into flower sales. Imagine my delight: flower bulb companies are now prepared to help schools raise funds by turning children into daffodil sellers instead of candy vendors. I heard a rumour that there are now 'sugar free' aisles in some American supermarkets.

A good start
Aerro's eating story from his mother:

'I knew that I wanted Aerro to start out with a good strong nutritional base. I knew for this to happen I wanted him to get a taste for vegetables rather than sweets. I heard that if babies are introduced to sweet foods first, they refuse vegetables. I think his first food other than breast milk was at four or five months. He was given diluted fresh vegetable juice in a bottle (carrot and celery). He loved it. Then I gave him mixtures of vegie and apple juice. His first solid food was steamed vegies mushed up. Then mushed banana.

'As his teeth started to come in he got more solid foods, but always cooked grains (he loves rice) or mushed vegies or mushed fresh fruit. When he started teething more he was made very happy by crackers to chew on. I gave him plain crackers without sugar and little salt, like rice cakes, rice crackers or Ryvita. I have found to this day he is always happy to eat simple foods. Toast with no butter, plain crackers and vegies with no salt (although he likes stir-fry with soy sauce or noodle and vegie soup with flavour). He has been exposed to cheese flavoured chips, the joy of cookies and other goodies. He loves those too, and his eyes light up when he sees a junk food packet. But he will still at two years old happily eat plain steamed vegies and rice, and loves fresh fruit.

'He was never given cow's milk at home. But he loves goat's yoghurt and sometimes goat cheese. The occasional times he has gotten a bit of cow's milk or cheese I immediately see him with a runny nose for a day or two. I have noticed one other thing. Where normally he wouldn't eat alfalfa sprouts, one time we were out and had only hot chips for lunch. I went and bought a container of alfalfa sprouts to eat with it, as I feel sick eating only greasy food. Well, Aerro asked for and ate up a good amount of those sprouts. I know he normally wouldn't but I felt that he knew on some level he wanted that green to help his tummy with the grease.

'I have noticed a big difference from other kids who were brought up on manufactured baby foods which are full of sugar and salt. These mothers with one year-olds with spotty faces remark on how healthy Aerro looks and how healthy his skin looks. These children also seem to be very picky about what they eat. They only want food with tons of flavour, salty or sweet. Many parents are amazed when they see Aerro eating exactly what I eat, instead of special food prepared for a picky child. I know he will be exposed to and probably eat lots of unhealthy food in his life. But I am very happy to know that he will happily and of his own choice eat healthy food as well.'

Emotional Healing for sugar freaks

Use the Melting Beachballs technique to find a way out of the sugar addiction and apathy maze.

Some familiar thought and word patterns

I can't see anyway	I 'm able to see
I'm too tired	I 'm full of energy
I don't matter	I'm important
I learned it but I can't use it	I use everything
I'd rather just sit here	I love to move

Put the words, 'I can't see' in your right hand Beachball. We'd better get a bicycle pump for this one. Getting enthusiastic about apathy is hard. You feel like you're encased in a heavy, lead diving-suit. Let's go diving then. The Beachball which says 'I can't see' is getting heavier and heavier and bigger. It's carrying you down and down into the dark mud. Here we are. How does it feel? Is it OK to be sunk in apathy, **in the can'ts**: 'I can't do, can't see, can't breathe, can't move' ? Can you give yourself a teeny ray of light down here? Think about it. Imagine it. Yes?

Let's ask ourselves, 'What is the opposite of 'I can't see'? 'You're able to see'? Is that OK too? That Beachball in your left hand is getting bigger. You're blowing it up with the bicycle pump? With your lungs? It's going to be tricky bringing that heavy lead ball and the airy light ball together. You'll find a way? Wonder-full! Now sing the song on page 219 with great enthusiasm.

Chapter Nineteen

Your child's room

Room designs and furnishings can remind, inspire and entice children to do vision games when they are alone. Place your home-made vision charts in strategic places; put nature posters and infinity signs over desks where school work is done.

Lighting, computers, homework

Fluorescent lighting - even when it is the new 'broad spectrum' lighting - still flickers at a frequency which is disturbing to the human organism. It has been shown to promote myopia. For these reasons I recommend incandescent or halogen light bulbs.

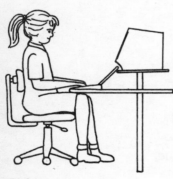

The light should fall directly downward onto yourchild's work or come from the side. The computer screen should be placed against a wall. If there is a light source from a lamp or window behind the screen, eye strain results. Your child's eyes are attracted to the light source even when his mind is trying to stay on the screen.

Right *Wrong*

Keeping your Magic Paintbrush moving across the computer screen will help prevent the development of 'computer eyes'. Paint the background colour of the screen with the Paintbrush. A wonderful habit for computer users to get into is Palming at the work station.

Prop your elbows on the desk and Palm for several seconds while the hard drive is making its manoeuvres. Moving your attention near and far flexes the muscles of accommodation. The NVI poster with eagle and crocodile provides a long road for Near-Far Swings at your desk. This poster features six vision games, including Painting White and Counting Cactus.

Ergonomics, the study of the relationship between workers and their environment, dictates that when using a computer, both feet should be on the floor and the spine erect. Hands and forearms on keyboards need to make a 90° angle with upper arms and shoulders. The Occupational Health and Safety Unit in Australia recommends a break from computer work every 15 minutes. If your child spends hours glued to a video or computer screen, work out a plan with him to do any of the vision games from this book at 15 to 30 minute intervals.

Design a vision nest for eaglets

The following room designs were devised during a Vision Improvement Playcamp, for children and their parents, held at the community house of Crystal Waters Permaculture Village. Optometric reports and life histories for the children were sent to us before the playcamp started.

During the five days of the camp we played vision games together, tailoring them to different ages and eyesight problems. Emotional Healing sessions were held first with parents, who were over-controlling their children's play. After releasing the pressure that their kids must exactly obey and instantly see better, we all relaxed.

The last day of the camp the children and teachers drew up room plans. We decided where the theme eyecharts would go on the wall, where the trampoline would be put and what rug they could lie on for Palming.

The following examples are all by hyperopic children. A room designed for a myopic child would be similar except that a young myope needs vistas. A Bug and Bead Game attached to a windowsill would allow him to take fusion and Near-Far Swings outwards into the landscape. Posters of oceans, skylines and mountain ranges could decorate his walls, providing settings for long-range visual journeys.

Jack's room (age eight)

The design team asked a number of questions, which were repeated for each child. Jacks history was considered first.

Jack's mother believed his brain damage had been caused by a triple antigen vaccination at six months. His left brain was affected, resulting in partial lameness on the right side of his body. Jack had a lazy left eye and had gone through two sets of prescriptions glasses for hyperopia to use at school. He refused to do eye exercises. 'He was sick of all the doctors,' his mother reported. In November of 1993 an optometrist had measured his vision at +2.25 with -0.50 x 180° axis. A paediatric ophthalmologist in October 1993 had measured Jack's vision at +6.75 with -2.00 x 10° and +7.25 with -1.5 at 175° axis. Just before coming to the Vision Playcamp, Jack had expressed, in the words of his mother, 'dissatisfaction with his physical drawbacks'.

Q. Teachers, what are the important games for Jack to play?

A. He needs lots of movement for hyperopia and Patching to bring his left eye outward. Use the Bug and Bead Game to solidify the fusion he achieved during Playcamp fusion games, plus lots of Cross-Crawling activities for his brain.

Q. Jack, what are your favourite vision games ?

A. Ball games and crawling games.

Q. What sort of ball games?

A. Soccer and football.

At home Jack shared a room with his two younger sisters while his parents were building an extension. The room we drew with Jack on a huge piece of paper looks like this.

Jack's room

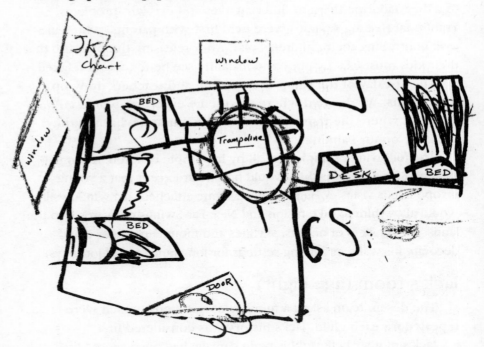

Daniel's room (age six)

The history report from Daniel's mother told us that he had a brain seizure in August of 1989 and was revived by ambulance staff. He had glasses for hyperopia since his vision problem was picked up by the pre-school nurse. His lenses had been strengthened three times. He was reversing some letters and his mum said his handwriting was terrible. An eye surgeon had measured Daniel's vision at +6.00 and +7.00. In February 1994 a behavioural optometrist

◉ Help Your Child to Perfect Eyesight

measured his eyes at +5.50 and +5.50. She sent me a thorough, typed visual assessment for the Playcamp. She found Daniel had no depth perception up close, and that with his glasses on his convergence was good.

Q. Teachers, what are the important vision games for Daniel to play?

A. As a hyperope Daniel needs his left brain switched on and movement to break the stare, especially up close. He loves the Ball on the String, and the Bug on the Bead. He uses a Halo when he does his Birds of a Feather Swing to increase saccadic movement.

Q. Daniel, what do you like most in your life?

A. Viruses: Daniel had watched a TV programme on viruses. He loves viruses. Therefore you have the privilege of seeing Daniel's renderings of viruses in this book.

Six weeks after the Playcamp: 'Daniel is no longer dependent on glasses. When his T-Glasses broke he put on his old prescription. They gave him headaches and sore eyes. He is doing most of the activities on most days and lots of Cross-Crawling. His handwriting has improved after working with an Edu-K counsellor'. His mother, Mandy, introduced the Magic Ribbon Wand to the First Grade class at their public school, with the principal's approval. The principal had to try it out himself first. Mandy is pleased with Daniel's progress. Daniel is happy.

Flash News Report: just before this manuscript goes to press I wish to add the most up-to-date report from Mandy. 'Whom can I tell? I am so excited and fired up. We've really achieved something.' I ask, 'Please tell me slowly, Mandy, what happened?' 'Because you had called and asked how Daniel was going, I took him back to the optometrist sooner than I had

Daniel's room

little 'virus' chart

Big 'Virus' chart

no people allowed

glasses in case (bye)

BEAD ON A STRING

Lightbulb

FOR HALO

SWINGING BALL ON STRING

cross-crawl MACHINE

mini-tramp

planned. She tested him and smiled. "Very nice changes in both eyes," she said. He was reading two lines better on the visual acuity test. He was passing the first test in depth perception. And his vision measured at +3.25 in both eyes. That's less than his original preschool prescription of +4.00 and +3.75.'

'Which activities have you been doing?' I asked.

'He's using the Swinging Ball right now. He uses his pin-holes on the computer. We do lots of Cross-Crawling. He's almost seven and he will do these things without being nagged. His Magic Ribbon Wand is around here somewhere.'

I asked to speak with Daniel to get the story from the lion's mouth. 'I've been doing that Ball Swing for a long time. Mummy does a sneaky Cross-Crawl with one finger and one toe.' When I asked Daniel how his viruses were doing, he said, 'I hate nightmares.' I suggested that when he sees a scary image in his dream that he assert, 'This is my dream, what are you doing here?'

Leanne's room (age nine)

Leanne joined the CHILDVISION Playcamp accompanied by her mother Yvonne. She had been prescribed glasses six weeks previously by a behavioral optometrist. There was a delay in obtaining her diagnosis on paper. Her mother had not understood the jargon used by the optometrist. In the meantime, Yvonne decided to experience NVI rather than rely solely on glasses to fix the problem. During the camp Leanne went without spectacles as she practiced all the basic games for hyperopia. She filled her bedroom design with vision games.

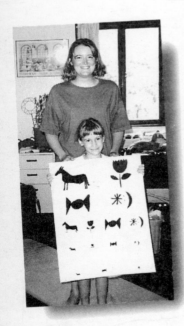

Leanne and her Janet Goodrich Method teacher Lynne Sheppard

Q.   Teachers, what vision games are important for Leanne?

A.   She needs Cross-Crawl and movement for hyperopia, Painting White for reading and the Bug and Bead game.

Q.   Leanne, what do you like?

A.   I like Sunning. I like birds and stars.

Six weeks after the Playcamp I received the original optometric report. The diagnosis was accommodative insufficiency. The recommended treatment was near (magnifying) spectacles of +0.75 for both eyes, as a training device. Secondly the optometrist wanted Leanne to take a course of in-office exercises with prisms. I explained to Yvonne that when Leanne looked alternately at far and close objects her ciliary muscles and hence the lens inside her eyes were not responding adequately. That's the accommodation aspect of her case. I suggested that Leanne, and her mother (who was feeling her own vision deteriorate from taking an advanced nursing course), do the Bug and Bead game at least twice a week. This would give Leanne some control over her own 'exercise' programme and flex both her accommodation and fusion.

Yvonne's follow-up report was that Leanne was doing Bird Swings and Palming; and her schoolteacher was letting her Palm in class. 'I took her back to the optometrist right after your course and he found her eyes had improved. He asked me what we had been doing.'

Leanne's room

I interviewed Leanne, who related, 'When I first started to forget to wear my glasses, when I put them on again, it goes all blurry.' To my question: 'What vision games are you doing and when?' Leanne replied, 'I'm using Palming a fair bit... like my eyes go all tired and they want to rest. It's a bit like when you wake up in the morning. Normally I think about snow. I see a white bunny go by, a house, a white bed, a ball, maybe a white pillow somewhere. Normally I feel pretty good if I do it that much. Then my eyes feel really good.'

Outdoor play areas

All children need time outdoors. After sedentary, mental games indoors, send everyone outdoors for raucous romping. At CHILD VISION Playcamps every child has equal indoor and outdoor time. All the Natural Vision Improvement games in this book can be played outdoors. To add to the challenge we set up par courses for children to run, with and without eye patches. This simple equipment can be easily set up at home or school. Leave the equipment standing so children can hone their motor and vision skills when no one is watching.

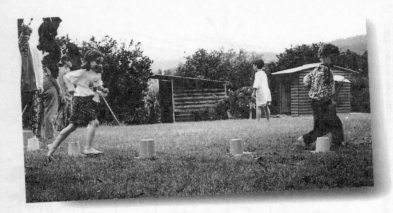

Margo and Daniel run the snake

Make crawling spaces from chairs and tables.

Secure old tyres set in wooden brackets to crawl through.

Set up traffic cones for running figure eights and snake patterns. We made traffic cones out of pink and yellow plastic flower pots. The pots can be tacked to a square piece of plywood to keep them stable.

Make a walking board. All children love to walk along cliffs. The safest cliff is a walking board. One sturdy long plank placed on two thick blocks of wood will suffice.

Use garbage bins for 'touch goals' and 'safe areas'.

For more ideas on developing perceptual and motor skills for use at home consult Jack Capon's book 'Perceptual-Motor Lesson Plans, Levels 1 and 2'.

If you'd rather have a folkloric, right-brain list of children's games, find 'Carmen Out to Play, A Collection of Children's Playground Games', compiled by Heather Russell. This book includes a number of games children teach one another: Colours Hopscotch, Mother May I?, Five Stones and Fortune Teller. The rules for these games are never fixed.

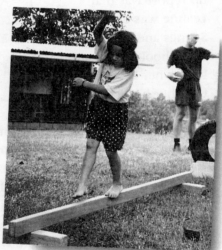

Margot walks the plank

Chapter Twenty

The hazardous classroom
History of western schooling

Schooling in the USA formed a model for the world. Academic methodology was based on the ideals of Benjamin Rush (1745-1812), chemist, social reformer and the most famous physician of his time. NVI teacher and sociology professor Raymond Welch made the following comments on Rush's plans for the American school child:

> 'In Rush's mind, schooling in the new Republic should be an advanced form of preventive social therapy. Almost all theorists and social planners of that age, European and American, agreed with Rush that the first concern of public schooling was not the formal subject matter as such, but the character of the young citizen. The moulding of good citizens became and remains the basic goal of the public school.'

This presumes the taming of spontaneous urges and the creation of a tractable, conservative and respectable youngster, a young citizen given to punctuality, discipline and order.

In Rush's ideal school, children were assigned small, fixed rectangular desks, arranged in rows. The drills for the day were to be strictly governed by allotted time segments and consisted of memorisation and recitation. In his essays Rush decreed that future generations were to be fitted into institutions laid down in the present: the masses were to be taught to acquiesce to the plans of the leaders. Schools were to replace the moral and social power of churches in colonial America and Europe.

As democracy spread through Europe and more freedom was given to the common person, a system for controlling that freedom was set in place.

In 1990 optometrist Raymond Gottlieb, who had improved his own sight with the Bates Method, described myopia in the 'Brain-Mind Bulletin' as the 'suppression of spontaneous urges.'

Before you think I'm putting all the blame for vision problems on the poor old school system, let me firmly state that social structures remain intact only through our acquiescence and cooperation. This gives us as parents the power to change schooling and what happens for our children in classrooms.

New hazards for old

Schools have changed, I am told. They are not as rigid as they used to be. Why then are more children developing vision problems as soon as they go to school? On the other hand, books such as 'The Learning Revolution' by Gordon Dryden and Jeannette Vos remind us that 'the home is the most important educational institution in the land'. Fifty percent of a person's ability to learn is developed in the first four years of life and another 30 percent by age eight. Carl Doman's book 'Teach Your Baby to Read' has inspired many parents to flash reading cards in the cradle. Myopia at age four, instead of age seven, may be the result.

Children are slaves to the ambitions of parents and governments. The first schools were free. Not free in the sense of paying money but free in the sense that you did not have to go. When schooling became compulsory until age 15 in many English speaking countries, some parents revolted, so did some teachers. Home schooling began; and alternative schools were set up.

Consider the Rudolf Steiner philosophy of child-raising. Every child develops in distinct phases. Left-brain scholastics out of phase with natural growth steal life energy from the child. The result is weakness and vulnerability to stress later in life. Steiner-oriented schools provide low-key environments for children to explore at their own pace. Music, art, wooden toys, poetry and rhymes are the modes through which science and maths are explored. A German survey showed that Steiner school graduates do well at university while maintaining humanitarian inclinations.

My daughter attended three different kinds of schools in her academic training period. The first was based on the values of Wilhelm Reich and of A.S. Neill, founder of the Summerhill School in England. The second, called Westland, was imbued with the notions of John Dewey - the 'hands on' learning man. We then ran out of alternative possibilities, and she entered public school for secondary education. Cybele shares her experience in alternative and regular schools:

'I remember playing a lot at Gateway. We were always doing something, engaging in some sort of exploration. This would be punctuated by a voice calling out that reading was happening, or maths, and everyone would go running; it was where the action was. The learning often took place in a circle on the floor, everyone taking turns. We put on plays from Dr Seuss and other books. It was fantastic.

'Later at Westland the curriculum was more regimented. Each class had a certain theme to explore. Grade threes were Harbour Masters. Grade fours were American Pioneers. Grade fives were Mexicans and Shopkeepers. With each theme we found ourselves pretending to be the characters we were learning about. This was done through crafts, food, clothing, plays, and a final presentation at the end of the semester to our parents. As Shopkeepers in grade five, we all took turns selling paper and other supplies to all the other grades. When I think back on the idea of the six and seven year-old class treasurers, lists in hand, going to ten year-olds to buy tempera paint, I smile.

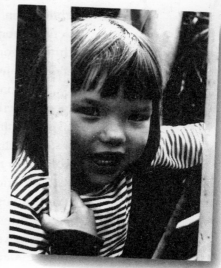

Cybele, three years old, at Gateway School

'Year six was my first year at a public school. My first of dreading school; and my first physical fight. Year eight I went to a private college preparatory school; They provided us with coffee and donuts every morning; well, orange juice and milk too. I later attended a number of different secondary schools but even the 'alternative' ones left me feeling cheated by a lack of joy in learning I had experienced earlier in my education. I didn't find it again at university either.'

Posture and seeing

A child's body is pliable and will mould itself to an unsuitable desk. Desks stay rigid like a pair of glasses, young bodies collapse into habitual slumps. Harmon's study caused school designers to throw out the big tables that children of all sizes had to adapt to. They were replaced by individual chairs because children do not come in the same packaging. Yet posture is still a problem when sitting at a computer as many adults have learned from the pain between the shoulder blades.

Good posture can be encouraged in several ways. Firstly pay attention to the furniture and lighting situation in the classroom and

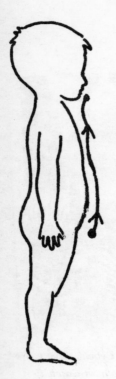

The central meridian

at home. The second area is energetic and emotional. When a child feels defeated and a failure because she is either zipping ahead of everyone else or lagging behind in the standards set for all the children in the grade, then we get a failure or frustration posture. The central meridian energy flow collapses. The thoughts running through your child's mind when sitting humped over her mid-line is 'I'm a failure'. The opposite is 'I'm a success'.

The command 'Sit up straight!' is a shock to the nervous system. More effective is a discussion about the child's attitude toward life. Using Melting Beachballs to resolve success and failure feelings can restore a child's central meridian flow. Central meridian energy runs from earth to sky, filling both right and left hemispheres of the brain with life energy. You can also use your hand to scoop up earth energy and bring up the mid-line of your body to restore joy and confidence. Simply bring your hand from groin to chin three times in a row, imagining your hand is full of flowing vital energy.

The Alexander Technique was devised by F M Alexander, an actor from Tasmania. After losing his voice on the Shakespearean stage, Alexander stopped acting and studied his own postural habits. By watching himself in a mirror he realized that every time he started to speak he raised his head slightly, effectively constricting his vocal cords. Alexander teachers can be found in many countries. Their work releases body energy in relationship to eyes. My first vision student in LA was Alexander instructor Judith Stransky. I gave her vision lessons and she helped with my posture. It was a mutually beneficial trade. If your child is slumping or her shoulders are rigid and high, Alexander lessons could restore her free and natural stance.

Emotional Healing for going to school

The general word/thought patterns for school are:

I'm a success   I'm a failure

Use the energy Beachballs. Put the statement 'I'm a failure' in your right hand. Give that ball a colour and a size and a weight. Repeat the words 'I'm a failure' in lots of different ways: sad, angry, don't-care-anyway or scared, until you can celebrate it and feel the love streaming toward you even when you are a failure. (Sometimes you are.)

When you are satisfied and have broadcast your message of 'I'm a failure' over hill and dale, ask what is the opposite of 'I'm a failure.' You may come up with a different sentence from mine. Maybe you have 'I can do anything' or 'I'm a genius'. Put whatever statement

👁 Help Your Child to Perfect Eyesight

you wish into your left hand. Turn it into a giant energy ball - or a tiny glowing magical gleaming energy ball made of titanium and gold. Announce and explore this thought until you think your two Beachballs somehow equal each other.

Melt, dissolve, squish the two balls together. Bring your hands to your heart and release the matter. Have a wonderful time learning in your own way, even if you have to go to school.. You may come to love school as you expand your capacity to love everything in your life.

Some parents have told me that their child is intensely competitive. Being competitive used to mean desiring success in the world. Times have changed. Stress in the business world results in personalities who make a lot of money and die young of heart attacks. Big business is now looking for teamwork and cooperation rather than 'get ahead of the competition' personalities. Human survival now requires practiced and automatic cooperation.

Competitive thought patterns derive from not accepting oneself as a significant being in a supportive universe. A competitive attitude results in a fighting stance, even in the shower. Trapezius and neck flexors never let go. Constant competition reverses the governing meridian. To help your child release a competitive stance and rock-hard shoulders, do Melting Beachballs with the following thought and word patterns:

I have to compete with others   I accept myself just as I am

A great day for eyes at school

Could all schools be better for children? Could going to school actually help children develop excellent eyesight instead of poor eyesight? This possibility is a movie in my mind starring Janet Goodrich Method teacher Phil McManus and his daughter Emma:

Hello Emma, what did you do at school today?

'In the morning we went outdoors and Sunned our eyes for a little while. Then we played ball. Catch. At first we were close together then we got farther and farther apart. Dad, I could catch a ball this tiny all the way from the end of the playing field. Without any glasses. I'll show you. Then we lay down in the grass while Margaret read us a story about an inventor. The guy who made aeroplanes. Kitty Hawk. That was the place. I remember it because we were Palming while Margaret read and when she said that place I made it into a cat and a bird in my mind.

Then we went inside. Michael gave us giant pieces of paper. We pasted them to the walls. I made lazy eights all over them to music.

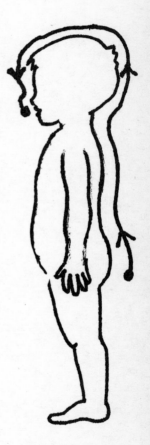

The governing meridian. Arrows show direction of life energy flow.

I can do hundreds of lazy eights. Look, I'll show you how in the dirt here. Lazy eights make a light go on in your head.

Tuesday we're going on a boat trip to watch the whales. We have some pictures to identify different seabirds and fish. So we hold the picture in our hands and do Near-Far Swings out to the birds. I'm going to see a dolphin. I can see them already in my head diving around. Sometimes they save people.

Did you know Dad, that when people are relaxed they can see better?

I'll go get some music and show you how to do the Cross-Crawl dance. I do it every time before my maths. It helps a lot. Put your right hand like this on your left knee...'

Children in the fast lane

Children either go for technology or reject it completely. A four year-old in Singapore who was once bright and rumbunctious sits listlessly in a chair after coming home from kindergarten. What doesn't he like about school? Children must learn to use a computer.

In Vancouver I see an eight year-old child daily glued to the screen, body hunched over his joystick, eyes engrossed in Nintendo. What are parents to do in these cases? The response must be individualised but it is obvious that in the first child a voice cries out, 'I don't want to be required to learn via a flat screen at my age.' The second child would probably scream bloody murder if his colour monitor were taken away. He says, 'This is the best thing in my life.'

Restriction, deprivation, caving in to cultural values: none of these policies 'from above' will have a beneficial effect. Parents will need to get more involved in the life of their child, internally and externally. They may need to change their own values. Parents definitely must make their own choices based on awareness of their child's needs, the possibilities available and what best fosters health and happiness.

Until now, parents have been cooperating in the creation of a myopic culture. There is a fear that their child will not do well in school or not be able to read the blackboard from the back of the room. The phrase is 'Keep up!' with others, who are also trapped in the race. This behaviour on the part of parents can end up as the 'Hurry Sickness' from which modern suburban-ites are suffering. Parents over-rule their initial instinctive questioning of putting a child in glasses. Some parents even agree to the prescription of one-quarter of a diopter correction. This is the minimum curve that can be ground into a lens.

👁 Help Your Child to Perfect Eyesight

Parents make it happen

Challenges

To summarise, these are the areas that you face as parent or care-taker of a child with a pair of eyes:

- the patronising attitude of government and doctors
- your own fear that your child will somehow be crippled or hindered if her vision is not corrected immediately with an optical device

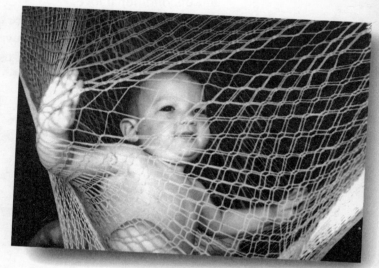

- the pressure of your peers and family members
- the fear of your child 'falling behind' in school
- your own lack of confidence
- your child's current dependence on glasses, either physical or emotional
- fear that your child may not take to the vision games, either because she is not inspired or (more often) because of negative associations with 'eye doctor stuff'.

The only way to escape being controlled by the above list is to realise that your love for children is all-powerful. Within you is still your initial gift of life energy. Bring out your inner child as a healing companion to your offspring. Give the child within yourself, and the child under your care, a chance to escape the trap!

Assets and support

Hold in your sights always the following:

- You are your own authority.
- Fear projects illusions into the future; fear is not reality.
- There is a universal healing force operative in your child.
- Confidence comes from experience. You don't have to know everything right now. Start with a baby step.
- Children will prefer not to use glasses once emotional ties and threats are removed.
- Vision games shared with enthusiasm are irresistible and effective.
- You will find professionals, friends and family members who will be supportive.

When you are down and it looks like nothing is working right, sing the next two songs. The Chinese Meridian Song combines self-encouragement, transmuting thought patterns and reviving energy flow through your whole body. Each statement in this song has an effect on the meridian noted and it's corresponding organ, body part or function.

The chant, Let This Child See, invokes the divine power of grace and unconditional love.

In the eyes of the child you see the origins of life. All superficial layers of conditioning are swept away in moments of joy. This is perfect sight, and it exists in every one of us!

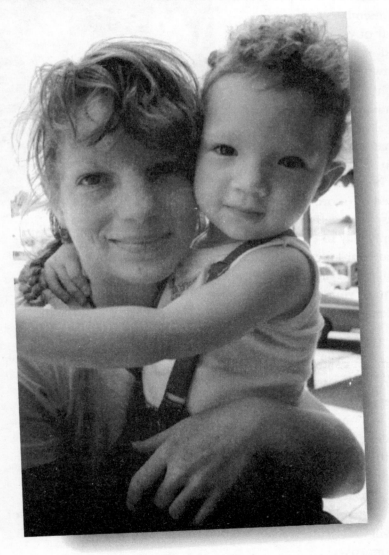

The Chinese Meridian Song

Music - Traditional
Words by Janet Goodrich

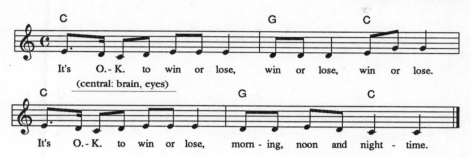

It's O.-K. to win or lose, win or lose, win or lose.

(central: brain, eyes)

It's O.-K. to win or lose, morn- ing, noon and night - time.

I accept me as I am, as I am, as I am… (governing: spine, ears)
It's O.K. to change and grow, change and grow, change and grow… (liver: change)
All my needs are satisfied, satisfied, satisfied… (stomach: digestion)
It's O.K. to look at me… (lung: shame, pride)
It's O.K. to see so far… (kidney: fear of life, love of life)
It's O.K. to see up close… (small intestine: assimilation, learning)
It's O.K. to fuse my eyes. (gall bladder: making choices)
I love seeing, yes I do… (heart: self-love)

Let This Child See

Words and melody by Janet Goodrich

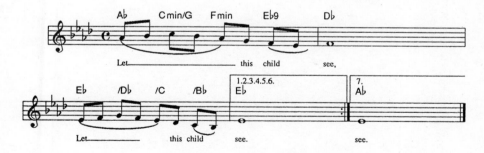

Let this child see,

Let this child see. see.

Definitions

ACCOMMODATION The ability of the visual system to see clearly distant and close.

ACCOMMODATION, MUSCLES OF (See CILIARY MUSCLE)

AMBLYOPIA (LAZY EYE) Reduced vision uncorrectable by glasses. It occurs when the brain 'switches off' the messages coming from a particular eye. This eye sometimes turns to one side or the other.

ARMOURING A word coined by Wilhelm Reich to describe chronic tightness of body muscles resulting from repression of emotional feelings. Armouring may manifest itself in eye muscles as well as in other parts of the body.

ASTIGMATISM Blurring of lines at a particular angle, caused by warping across the cornea and sometimes lens of the eye. Astigmatism comes and goes and is affected by stress, eye strain, posture and emotional factors.

AUTONOMIC NERVOUS SYSTEM The part of our nervous system that functions automatically and is in charge of maintaining a stable internal environment.

BATES METHOD Techniques for relaxing and mobilising the whole visual system devised by American ophthalmologist William H Bates. This method emphasized the connection between the body and mind and gave individuals a way to improve their sight without depending on glasses.

BEHAVIOURAL OPTOMETRY A specialized branch of optometry which recognizes the influence of environment, posture and general health on eyesight. The treatment is a combination of training lenses and eye exercises.

BILIRUBIN The red/yellow pigment found in bile, blood and urine.

CATARACT A pathological eye disease in which the lens of the eye is clouded.

CHI The Chinese term for universal life energy.

CHIROPRACTIC A system of healing based upon the theory that disease results from a lack of normal nerve function. Treatment consists of manipulation and specific adjustments of body structures, especially the spinal column.

CILIARY MUSCLE The muscle which encircles the lens of the eye. It contracts and releases, changing the shape of the lens thus producing accommodation.

CONE CELLS Specialised nerve cells on the retina which produce colour and detail vision.

CONCAVE LENSES a lens which curves inward, used to compensate for myopia. This lens makes things look smaller.

CONVEX LENSES a lens which curves outward, used to compensate for hyperopia. This lens magnifies.

CORNEA The transparent front of the eye that covers the iris and pupil.

CORPUS CALLOSUM An area of the brain composed of neural fibres which interconnect the hemispheres. This 'bridge' between the hemispheres allows them to share memory and learning and to work together.

CROSS-CRAWL A remedial self-help action which reaffirms the bilateral patterning laid down during the crawling stage of infancy. This action combines physical movements requiring simultaneous input from both the left and right hemispheres of the brain. Through this movement both sides are stimulated, 'switched on' and brought to work together.

DIOPTER The measurement unit used for describing refractive error on prescriptions. One diopter is the refractive power of a lens needed to focus a point of light at one metre's distance.

DIVERGENCE Moving away from a central point or line. A term used to describe eyes that turn outward. (See STRABISMUS)

DNA (DIOXYRIBONUCLEIC ACID) An acid found in cells which assists in the transfer of genetic information.

DOMINANT Commanding or controlling. This term is used to describe the sides of the brain and body which are used first, ie each individual is either right or left brain dominant, dictating their particular tendancies even when they are using both sides. (See RIGHT & LEFT BRAIN.) A 'right-handed' individual can be described as 'right hand dominant'.

DYSLEXIA A state in which an individual has 'switched off' part of his abilities, usually due to stress or trying too hard. This may result in slow reading, reversal of letters when writing, or disruption of personal expressiveness.

EMMETROPIA Normal refractive condition of the eye.

ENZYMES Chemicals created by living cells that catalyse processes in the body. The most well known enzymes are those used by the body for digesting foods. Digestive enzymes are essential for the breaking down of foods into their nutrient components for use by the body.

ESOTROPIC This describes an eye that turns inward (cross-eyed) (See PHORIA).

EXOTROPIC This describes an eye that turns outward (wall-eyed). (See PHORIA)

FOVEA CENTRALIS The point of keenest vision in the eye, located inside the macula lutea. In this area a very large number of cone cells are massed tightly together. When light enters the lens and is cast directly on the fovea centralis, sharp, detailed images will result.

FOVEAL VISION Sharp, clear vision acheived by the fovea centralis. Also called 'nuclear' and 'central' vision. (See NUCLEAR VISION).

FUSION The brain and mind's ability to create one image from the messages coming from both eyes.

FUSIONAL RESERVE A reserve of strength and energy in the visual system which allows clear vision and fusion to take place through periods of strain. This reserve lasts for a certain period and can be 're-charged', but will not be maintained through long periods of constant stress.

'GATE' The appearance of two fingers that arises when one finger is held up close in front of the eyes and the attention is in the distance. This double-image shows that fusion is happening in the visual system.

GLAUCOMA A pathological eye disease characterised by abnormal fluid pressure within the eyeball.

'GREAT WHITE GLOW' The white aura seen around letters and words when viewing black print on white paper with a relaxed mind.

HEMISPHERE The right half or left half of the brain.

HOMOLATERAL Using only one side of the brain or body. This can result in an inability to perform creatively, express spontaneously and maintain health. Homolateral movement is the opposite of the 'Cross-Crawl'.

HYPEROPIA (LONG-SIGHTEDNESS) A state in which images of close objects fall behind the retina rather than on it, resulting in visual blur. The physical aspect is an abnormally short eyeball. The emotional aspect is discomfort with closeness, intimacy, details. Usually compensated for by prescribing of magnifying or 'plus' lenses.

INTEGRATION The merging and blending of abilities and characteristics. The act of unifying rather than isolating. Denotes a state of high human ability.

JAUNDICE A yellowish discolouration of the skin, mucous membranes and body fluids caused by an excess of bilirubin. Not uncommon in newborns, the most widely known remedy is placing the infant in direct sunlight for short periods.

LEFT BRAIN The left hemisphere of the brain; its abilities and actions. These include counting, analyzing, verbalising, reasoning and trying.

LENS The transparent layered curved structure that sits between the pupil and vitreous humor. The lens gently bends entering light and helps bring it to a point on the retina.

LIFE ENERGY The universal creative force which brings all beings into life, which restores them to a state of balance and health when they go off track.

LYMPHATIC SYSTEM A major component of our immune system, the lymphatic system is composed of a clearish fluid which carries proteins, hormones and fats to all body cells. It carries toxins away from cells, produces antibodies and manufactures one quarter of our white blood cells. It is unlike the vascular system of blood transport in the body, which is moved by the action of the heart pumping the blood. Instead lymph fluid is pumped through the body by the movement of muscles.

LYMPHATIC BOUNCING Small gentle jumps on a mini-trampoline which create suffcient muscular movement and gravitational pull to move lymph fluid through the body.

MACULA LUTEA A small area on the retina in a direct line back from the lens of the eye. It has a higher concentration of the cone receptor cells than the rest of the retina.

MELANIN A pigment in human skin. It helps to protect the skin from over-exposure to sunlight.

MELATONIN A hormone which is stimulated by light. Melatonin affects the brain as well as other glands such as the adrenals, pituitary, testes and ovaries. It is also involved in regulating sleeping cycles. It may function as a stress hormone and can affect sexual development.

MINI-TRAMPOLINE A small trampoline often used indoors. These are available from a numbers of manufacturers and vary in price according to the quality. They usually measure approximately one metre (one yard) across.

MYOPIA (SHORT-SIGHTEDNESS) A state of the visual system in which images of distant objects fall in front of rather than on the retina, resulting in blur. Physically, the eyeball is too long. Emotionally, myopes usually have difficulty wanting to see or open up to the larger world. Usually compensated for by prescribing of contractive 'minus' lenses.

NATURAL VISION IMPROVEMENT — THE JANET GOODRICH METHOD A method of improving eyesight by wholistic means, without the use of optical devices. Comprised of the Bates Method creatively merged with principles of brain function, psychology, and general health, NVI combines working with the physical state of the visual system, the emotional and mental state of the individual, and lifestyle habits.

NEURO-LYMPHATIC The lymphatic system is part of the immune system of the body. Neuro-lymphatic reflexes and points are those relating to the interaction between the nervous and lymphatic systems.

NEURO-VASCULAR REFLEXES/POINTS Reflexes involving both nervous and vascular structures. (Nerves and blood vessels) Points located mainly on the head which stimulate and regulate parts of the nervous and vascular systems.

NUCLEAR VISION A term coined by Janet Goodrich to describe centralised, crystal clear foveal vision. Mentally the object regarded is seen more clearly than anything surrounding it. Physically the light from the object regarded falls into the fovea centralis. (See FOVEAL VISION).

OBLIGATION (as used in this book) The requirement to perform to a certain standard. In the case of eye tests, this 'obligation to perform' in itself creates a stressful situation which can result in visual blur.

OCULAR ANAESTHESIA Anaesthesia used on the eye so that surgery can be performed.

OPTIC CHIASM The intersection of the optic nerves from the two eyes. At this point in the brain the optic nerve fibres divide, half from each eye crossing over to join half from the other eye.

OPHTHALMOLOGIST A medical doctor specializing in examining eyes and prescribing glasses, diagnosing and treating eye diseases. Performs optional surgeries for strabismus and myopia.

OPTOMETRIST Examines eyes and prescribes glasses. Diagnoses but usually refers eye diseases. Behavioural optometrists also give eye exercises.

ORTHOPTICS A medically accepted method of exercising eye muscles to correct crossed eyes and muscular weakness. Commonly used for a short period after surgery.

OSTEOPATH A practitioner of osteopathy.

OSTEOPATHY A system of medical treatment based on the theory that diseases are chiefly due to the loss of structural integrity in the tissues of the body. Treatment consists of body manipulation (adjustments) surgery, drugs, and diet.

PALMING Gently placing the cupped palms of the hands over closed eyes to relax by visualising pleasant images.

PATCHING Covering one eye with an obscuring material to encourage the uncovered eye to wake up, perceive and strengthen.

PHORIA The tendency of lines of vision to deviate from the normal. Esophoria is the tendency of eyes to deviate (turn) inward (towards the nose). Exophoria is the tendency of eyes to deviate in an outward direction.

PHORIA, FAVOURING THE Referred to when playing vision games. The turning eye is stimulated to resume a normal line of vision, opposite the direction that the eye is turning.

PITUITARY GLAND The body's 'concertmaster' which secretes hormones that regulate the endocrine system.

PTERYGIUM A fleshy mass of conjunctiva which usually occurs at the inner side of the eyeball, covering part of the cornea. Pterygiums can cause a disturbance of vision by growing across the pupil.

REFLEX A physical movement or internal change performed automatically and without conscious volition. Nerve impulses sent from various parts of the body are received by the brain, which sends back an instant and automatic response. There are several different kinds of reflexes in the human body. The important ones for healing are messages passed between muscular, organ, and nerve systems.

REFLEX POINT A small area in a specific location on the body. When stimulated these points send information and energy to the relevant organ, muscles or nerve system which helps in activating and regulating their function.

REFRACTIVE ERROR A deviation in the eye's ability to bend incoming light to create a clear image. Variations are labeled as hyperopia, myopia, presbyopia ('old-age sight') and astigmatism.

REICHIAN THERAPY A method of changing human unhappiness by freeing breathing patterns and increasing the flow of biological energy through the body. Values that are part of Reichian principles include natural childbirth, self-regulation and self-responsibility, positive sexual and emotional expression and human autonomy.

REM (RAPID EYE MOVEMENT) Prior to going into deep sleep an individual's eyes make many rapid small movements behind closed lids.

RETINA The responsive layer of specialised nerve cells at the back of the eye which change light into electrical impulses.

RETINOSCOPE An optical instrument that casts a beam of light into the eye revealing whether it is in a state of refractive error.

RETINOSCOPY Objective examination of the refractive powers of the eye by observation with a retinoscope.

RIGHT BRAIN The right hemisphere of the brain; its abilities and actions. These include rhythmic movement through space, imaging, musicality, and supplying balanced energy to all body muscles.

ROD CELLS Nerve cells in the retina which register light and dark. They are stimulated in dim light and do not register colour.

SACCADES Quick, small movements that enable the eyes to pick up details and to move from one object of interest to another.

'SEASONAL AFFECTIVE DISORDER' (SAD): An affliction suffered by people who live in areas of long winters, with short daylight periods. A lack of sufficient light (sunlight) causes depression and malaise.

SELF-REGULATION A principle used in child-centred schooling and nurturing. Children determine their own activities and schedules. Best understood as meaning freedom, not licence.

SQUINT (See STRABISMUS)

STRABISMUS Turning of an eye so that both eyes are unable to look at the same point simultaneously.

SUNNING Relaxing for short periods in the sunlight with eyes closed. Sunning allows body and eyes to absorb the small amount of UV light essential to human health.

SWING Moving attention and body to relax and to activate rapid saccadic movement in the eyes.

'TOUCH FOR HEALTH' A system for lay people to correct and restore body energy using muscle testing. Pressure points on the body are activated to improve posture, relieve headaches, indigestion and other ailments before the underlying imbalances result in disease.

TRANSITION ('T') GLASSES Under-corrected glasses worn by Natural Vision Improvement students which give eyes room for change and allow the student to see adequately when necessary.

TROMBONING Covering one eye with the palm and moving an object near and far to strengthen and flex the components of accommodation.

ULTRA-VIOLET (UV) That part of the sun's rays with slightly greater frequency than violet. It is also emitted by artificial lamps that are used for healing, growing plants and forming vitamins. Ultra-violet is said to be necessary for human health as it stimulates the pituitary gland.

VISUAL CORTEX A part of the cerebral cortex in the brain, primarily responsible for interpreting visual impulses from the eyes. Also called the visual brain.

WHOLISTIC The person is regarded as a whole being made up of physical, emotional, mental and spiritual components. In healing, the opposite of regarding symptoms in isolation.

References
(in order of mention)

Chapter One

Reich, Wilhelm *Selected Writings, An Introduction to Orgonomy* The Noonday Press 1973

Duke-Elder, Sir Stewart *The Practice of Refraction* (7th edition) J & A Churchill Ltd 1963

Huxley, Aldous *The Art of Seeing, An Adventure in Re-education* Harper & Brothers New York & London 1942

Bates, WH *The Bates Method for Better Eyesight Without Glasses* Jove Publications Inc 1978

Lierman, Emily *Stories From The Clinic* New York 1926

Myopie Kann Nicht Trainiert Werden DVA 1989

Gesell, Arnold; Ilg, Frances & Bullis, Glenna *Vision: Its Development in Infant and Child* Paul B. Hoeber Inc New York 1949

Raknes, Ola *Wilhelm Reich and Orgonomy* Penguin Books 1971

Wertenbaker, Lael *The Eye: Window to the World* Torstar Books USA 1984

Mueller, Conrad G, Rudolph Mae & the editors of Time-Life Books *Light and Vision* Time-Life Books 1966

Manual of Ocular Diagnosis and Therapy (3rd edition) ed Deborah Pavan-Langston, MD Little, Brown & Company Boston MA USA 02108

Corbett, Margaret *Help Yourself to Better Eyesight* Prentice Hall 1949

The Myopia Epidemic Faye Hammel, New York Sunday News Magazine 220E 42nd St New York City 10017 May 18 1980

Thie, John F *Touch For Health* DeVorss & Co 1979 (published in Australia by Second Back Row Press Katoomba NSW 1984)

Harmon, Darell Boyd *The Co-ordinated Classroom* Booklet 1951

Yarbus, Alfred L *Eye Movements and Vision* Plenum Press New York 1967

Chapter Two

Myopia: Prevalence and Progression, Committee on Vision Commission on Behavioral and Social Sciences and Education National Research Council National Academy Press Washington DC 1989

Duke-Elder, Sir Stewart *The Practice of Refraction* (7th Edition) J & A Churchill Ltd London 1963

The Transmission of Refractive Errors Within Eskimo Families Young, FA, Leary, GA, Baldwin, WR & West, DC 1969 American Journal of Optometry 46 pp 676-685

20/20 Is Not Enough, Sekuler, Robert PhD and Mulvanny, Patrick PhD American Health Nov/Dec 1982

Psychological Changes in Bates Method Students LaSalle, Coralee unpublished dissertation UCLA 1975

Psychological Factors In Myopia Kelley, Charles R Journal Am. Optom. Assoc. 33(6): 833-837 1967

A comparative psychological investigation in myopes and emmetropes Van Alphen Proc, K, Nederl. Akad. Wet. 55 (5) 689-696 1951

Emmetropia and ametropia, In Refractive Anomalies NINDS Monograph 5 Subcommittee on Vision and Its Disorders, Bethesdaa, MD; US National Advisory Neurological Diseases & Blinding Council 1967

Reichian Therapy; The Visual Block Goodrich, J unpublished dissertation Antioch University Without Walls 1976

Chapter Three

Letter, House of Representatives Committee on Post Office and Civil Service May 11 1982 to Clinton R Miller, then Executive Director, National Health Federation Monrovia California 91076

Seeing Space, Undergoing Brain Re-programming To Reduce Myopia Orfield, Antonia OD *Journal of Behavioral Optometry* Vol 5 1994

Graeme Thompson ACBO 374 Pennant Hills Rd Pennant Hills NSW 2120 (personal communication)

Liberman, Jacob *Take Off Your Glasses and See* Crown Books 1994

Kavner, Richard S. OD *Your Child's Vision, A Parent's Guide to Seeing, Growing and Developing* New York 1985

Geoff Gillett, Medicare Program Branch, Health Insurance Commission, Tuggeranong ACT Australia

Flax, Nathan, OD and Duckman, Robert, OD, *Orthoptic treatment of Strabismus,* Journal American Optometric Association, Vol 49 Number 12

Chapter Five

Charles Handy Sees The Future, Rapoport, Carla Time Magazine 13 February 1995

Gesell, Arnold; Ilg, Frances L & Bullis, Glenna E Vision: *Its Development in Infant and Child* Paul B Hoeber Inc 1949

Geo Wissen Magazine Germany Nr 2/September 1993

Schell, Robert E and Hall, Elizabeth *Developmental Psychology Today* (4th edition) Random House Inc 1983

Magoun, Harold I. (Editor) *Osteopathy in The Cranial Field 2nd Edition* The Journal Printing Company USA 1966

Silverstein, Samuel *Child Spirit* Bear & Co Publishing Santa Fe NM 1991

Cameron Dawson 2 June 1995 (personal communication)

Chapter Six

Walther, David S *Applied Kinesiology Vol. 1 Basic Procedures and Muscle Testing Systems* DC Colorado USA 1981

Leboyer, Frederick *Loving Hands* Collins 1977

Chapter Seven

Fincher, Jack *The Brain, Mystery of Matter and Mind* US News Books Washington DC, 1981

Beware The Baby Walker, Consumers Digest January/February 1993

Dennison, Paul *Switching On, A Guide to Edu-Kinesthetics* Edu-Kinesthetics Inc Glendale California 1981

Schell, Robert E and Hall, Elizabeth *Developmental Psychology* Today (4th edition) Random House Inc 1983

Diamond, MC, Scheibel, AB, Elson, LM *The Human Brain Coloring Book* Harper & Row USA 1985

Chapter Eight

Fisher Sea, Jan *No Bored Babies: A Guide to Making Developmental Toys for Babies Birth-Age Two* Bear Creek Publications USA 1990

Bruna, Dick *The Fish* Follett Publishing Company 1963

Stern, John A *The Sciences* New York Academy of Sciences 1988

Yarbus, Alfred L *Eye Movements and Vision* Plenum Press New York 1967

Chapter Nine

Price Todd, Gary *Nutrition, Health & Disease* Whitford Press USA 1985

Liberman, Jacob *Light Medicine of the Future* Bear & Company Inc USA 1991

Ott, John N *Health and Light* Ariel Press USA 1976

Kime, Zane R *Sunlight Can Save Your Life* World Health Publications USA 1980

Hollwich, F The *Influence of Ocular Light Perception on Metabolism in Man and in Animal* Springer-Verlag NY Inc 1979

Samuels & Samuels *The Well Pregnancy Book* Summit Books 1986

Plain Common Sense vs. Scientific Theoretical Irrationality, The International Journal of Biosocial Research (Vol 7) Biosocial Publications PO 1174 Tacoma WA 98401

Chapter Ten

Martha J Farah *Is Visual Imagery Really Visual? Overlooked Evidence From Neuro-psychiatry* Psychological Review 95 pp307-317 1988

Mueller, Else *Traeumen auf der Mondschaukel Koesel* 1993

Chapter Eleven

Busacca, Richard *The Individual in Society & Culture* San Francisco State University

Krishnamurti, J *Krishnamurti to Himself* Victor Gollancz London UK 1987

Chapter Twelve

Yarbus, Alfred L *Eye Movements and Vision* Plenum Press New York, 1967

Chapter Thirteen

Gesell, Arnold; Ilg, Frances L & Bullis, Glenna E Vision: *Its Development in Infant and Child* Paul B Hoeber Inc 1949

Goodbye Glasses? Consumer Reports Harvard Medical School Health Letter January 1988 USA

Chapter Fifteen

Duke-Elder, Sir Stewart *The Practice of Refraction* (7th edition)
J & A Churchill Ltd 1963

Chapter Sixteen

Jacob, Stanley W & Francone, Clarice Ashworth *Structure and Function in Man* (3rd edition) WB Saunders Company USA 1974

Goodrich, Janet *Natural Vision Improvement* Viking Penguin 1990

Samuels, Mike MD & Nancy *The Well Baby Book* Summit Books USA 1991

Kavner, Richard S OD *Your Child's Vision, A Parent's Guide to Seeing,Growing and Developing* New York 1985

Duke-Elder, Sir Stewart *The Practice of Refraction* (7th edition)
J & A Churchill Ltd 1963

Cameron Dawson June 2 1995 (personal communication)

Chapter Seventeen

Jacob, Stanley W & Francone, Clarice Ashworth *Structure and Function in Man* (3rd edition) WB Saunders Company USA 1974

Chapter Eighteen

Dufty, William *Sugar Blues* Chilton New York 1975

Health Discoveries Newsletter Lafayette Institute for Basic Research Inc PO Box 6306 Charlottesville Virginia 22906 (804) 9732196

Milk, is it really good for you? Cutter, Karin. Well Being Magazine Sydney September 1995.

Chapter Twenty

Making a Spectacle World Welch, Raymond unpublished essay written during his training as an NVI teacher in Los Angeles 1981

Neill, AS *Summerhill A Radical Approach to Child Rearing* Hart Publishing Co New York 1960

Recommended reading

No Bored Babies: A Guide to Making Developmental Toys for Babies Birth-Age Two Fisher Sea, Jan, Bear Creek Publications USA 1990

Switch on Your Brain Parker, Allan & Cutler-Stuart, Margaret, Hale & Iremonger Pty Ltd Australia 1986

Carmen Out to Play! Russell, Heather, Oxford University Press 1989

Games for Growing Babies Crockford, Patricia, Bridgewater Books Australia 1989

Games for Growing Two Year Olds Crockford, Patricia, Bridgewater Books Australia 1989

Games for Growing Toddlers Crockford, Patricia, Bridgewater Books Australia 1989

Child Spirit. Children's Experience with God in School Silverstein, Samuel, Bear & Company Publishing USA 1991

Recommended nutrition & recipe books

Acquiring Optimal Health Price Todd, Gary, Hampton Roads Publishing Company Inc USA 1994

The Australian Family Vegetarian Cookbook Stephens, Helen, Hyland House Publishing Pty Ltd 1994

Raw Energy Recipes Kenton, Leslie & Susannah, Century Publishing Co Ltd London 1985

Healthy Food Your Kids Will Love! O'Dea, Jenny, Currey O'Neil Ross Pty Ltd Australia 1985

Healthy Cooking Stanton, Rosemary, Murdoch Books 1993

Recommended picture books for children

Level 1
Baby Says Pragoff, Fiona, Harper Collins Publishers Ltd 1994

The Fish Bruna, Dick, Follett Publishing Company 1963

Little Bird Tweet Bruna, Dick, Follett Publishing Company 1963

Level 2
Dear Zoo Campbell, Rod, Picture Puffins 1984

Rosie's Walk Hutchins, Pat, Picture Puffins 1970

Level 3
I Spy Fantasy, A Book of Picture Riddles Wick, Walter & Marzollo, Jean, Scholastic Inc 1994

The Junk Drawer Berrett, Rebecca, The MacMillan Company of Australia 1988

Harold and the Purple Crayon Johnson, Crockett, Harper Collins Publishers 1983

Wacky Wednesday LeSieg, Theo, Random House Inc 1974

The Bad-Tempered Ladybird Carle, Eric, Picture Puffins 1982

Each Peach Pear Plum Ahlberg, Janet and Allan, Picture Puffins 1989

Mr. Squiggle and the Preposterous Purple Crocodile Hetherington, Norman and Margaret, ABC Enterprises Australia 1993

Level 4

Imagine Lester, Alison, Allen and Unwin Pty Ltd Australia 1992

The Journey Home Lester, Alison, Oxford University Press 1990

For Eagle Eyes Only Heimann, Rolf, Periscope Press Australia 1993

Ultimaze Book Heimann, Rolf, Periscope Press Australia 1993

Where's Wendy? Tallarico, Anthony, Kidsbooks Incorporated USA 1991

Abigail goes visiting Pirani, Felix, Diamond Books London 1994

Where's Wally? 3 The Fantastic Journey Handford, Martin, Century Hutchinson Australia Pty Ltd 1990

Level 5

Whatley's Quest Whatley, Bruce & Smith, Rosie, Angus & Robertson Publication 1994

Animalia Base, Graeme, Puffin Books 1990

Willy and the Ogre Tonkin, Rachel, Hodder & Stoughton (Australia) Pty Ltd 1991

The Rainbow Goblins de Rico, Ul, Thames & Hudson Inc USA 1978

Magic Eye NE Thing Enterprises, Viking 1993

Recommended reading on Vision Improvement

Natural Vision Improvement Goodrich, Janet PhD
(available at all major bookshops or the NVI head office)

Publishers

Australia Penguin Books, Melbourne, VIC
USA Celestial Arts, Berkeley CA
Germany VAK Verlag, Freiburg
Spain Editorial Mirach, Madrid
France Terre Vivante, Paris
England Penguin Books, London

Take Off Your Glasses and See Liberman, Jacob
Crown Publishers Inc NY 1995

on Light

Sunlight Can Save Your Life
Kime, Zane MD
World Health Publications
PO Box 408 Penry CA 95663
Ph 916 8236655

Light, Medicine of the Future
by Liberman, Jacob OD, PhD
Word of Life Distributors   or   Universal Light Technology
FCTY 3 Lot 32 Industrial Ave   PO Box 4058
Somerville VIC 3912 Australia: Aspen CO 81612-4058 USA
Ph 059 776106

on Education

Greenberg, Daniel, *Sudbury Valley School, Free At Last*
Sudbury Valley School Press, #2 Winch St. Framingham, MA 01701 USA

Neill, A S, *Summerhill A Radical Approach to Child Rearing*
Hart Publishing Co 74 Fifth Ave New York NY USA
(by the same author: Freedom, Not License)

The Prepared Mind A reader-friendly magazine for parents, educators and students that explains current trends in learning, eg multi-age groupings, co-operative learning, accelerated learning, parent participation in schools. For subscription write to: *The Prepared Mind Network* PO Box 602, Kenmore, QLD 4069 Australia Ph (015) 745 620

Resources

Cassettes

Natural Vision Improvement album:
Janet Goodrich talks you through ten vision improvement activities plus seven colour stories. Original music on six audio cassettes.
Available only from certified teachers or the NVI head office:
The Janet Goodrich Method
12 Crystal Waters
MS 16 Maleny
QLD 4552 Australia

To purchase books by Jack Capon and for free catalogue of guidebooks for movement education and perceptual-motor development, write to:
Front Row Experience
540 Discovery Bay Blvd
Byron CA 94514-9454 USA

Children's motor development classes:
Toddler Kindy Gymbaroo
Parent/Child Education Centres
4 Selbourne Rd
Kew VIC 3101
Ph (03) 818 6927

Eye professionals & body workers

Australasian College of Behavioural Optometrists
374 Pennant Hills Road
Pennant Hills NSW 2120
ph (02) 481 0449

Jenny Livanos
Holistic Optometry Association
Shop 12 199 Beamish St
Campsie NSW 2194
Ph (02) 718-2951

Cameron Dawson Technologies
for the Dawson Programme
PO Box 45 Ocean Grove
VIC 3226
052 551396
1-800-64-8668

Alexander Technique, Australian Society of Teachers of the
16 Princes St
Kew
VIC 3101
Freecall (008)33-9571

Consult your local phone book for addresses of osteopathic and chiropractic associations.

To contact a practitioner of Touch for Health & Educational Kinesiology

Australian Kinesiology Association
PO Box 155
Ormond VIC 3204
Ph 03 578 1229

North American TFH Association
6955 Fernhill Drive
Malibu CA 90265
ph 310 457 8342

TFH Association of Canada
Box 74508
Kitsailano Postal Unit
Vancouver BC V6K 4P4
Ph 604 978 6292

The British Kinesiology Federation
30 Dudley Road
West Sussex PO21 1ER, England
Ph 243 841 689

TFH Association of NZ
33 Gilshennan Valley
Red Beach, New Zealand
Ph 9426 7695

Information on nutrition and eye pathologies

Dr Gary Price-Todd
Bio-Zoe Inc
PO Box 49
Waynesville NC 28786 USA
Ph (704) 452-0472
Fax (704) 456-4471

Dr. Lesley Salov
Vision & Health Center
W3064 Piper Road
Whitewater, WI 53190 USA
Ph (414) 473-7361

Index

👁 Help Your Child to Perfect Eyesight

Acknowledgments

I wish to thank Cybele, Carina and Aerro Goodrich-Harwell, my parents, childhood friends and teachers. Children at Crystal Waters Permaculture Village and surrounding area grace these pages with their bright eyes. Local musicians Don Woodward, Bernard O'Scanaill and Elizabeth Ledger gifted their music. Robin Harpley helped me with research. My husband Geraldo lent constant support on all fronts. Artists Veronica Davidson, Fiona Whipp, and Chris Dent brought words to life with images. I thank the optometrists and ophthalmologists who helped me with technical data. My heart-felt gratitude goes to Jill Morris, Amber, Dave, the Richardson family, Steve Wall and family, Elaine Wood, Grant Hammer, the children and parents at Playcamps, and especially the teacher trainees who relived their own childhood in the process of healing their sight.

My gratitude extends to the thousands of people who have had the courage and interest to receive, use and pass on a greater truth about vision.

Janet Goodrich

Alphabetical list of songs

<CHILDVISION> Teachers

The following Natural Vision Improvement instructors have completed both the basic training course with Janet Goodrich and supplementary studies in teaching children:

Joy Glengarry, 87 Monument St., Mosman Park, Western Australia, 6012. Phone: (09) 385-0565

Jean Ponchard, 2/3 Manion Ave., Rose Bay, New South Wales, 2029. Phone: (02) 371-6325

Betty Munro, 10 Margaret St., Devonport, Tasmania, 7310. Phone: (004) 24-8061

Grant Calvert, 1st Floor, 75 Archer St., Chatswood, New South Wales, 2067. Phone: (02) 411-7488

Lynne Hogg, 287 Boundary Rd., Maraylya, New South Wales, 2765. Phone: (045) 73-6121

Carina Goodrich, 12 Crystal Waters Vlg., MS 16, Maleny, Queensland, 4552. Phone: (07) 5494-4657

Michael van den Bergh, 25 Bellevue Ave., Salisbury, Queensland, 4107. Phone: (07) 3277-7856

Maria Gillanders, 1 Mather Rd, Yungaburra, Queensland, 4872. Phone: (070) 953-784, after Nov 1997 (07) 4095-3781

Ivan Sacher, 50 Athalie Ave., Linksfield, North Johannessburg, 2192, South Africa. Phone: (011) 640-6555

Contact the Janet Goodrich Centre for an updated list of <CHILDVISION> Teachers: 12 Crystal Waters Village, MS 16, Maleny, Queensland, 4552, Australia. Until October, 1996 the phone number is (074) 94-4657. After October 1996, the phone number is (07) 5494-4657.

Ask for information on trampolines, pin-holes, cassettes, books, seminars and training.

"Buy your own"

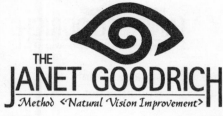

THE JANET GOODRICH
Method <Natural Vision Improvement>
VITALIZER

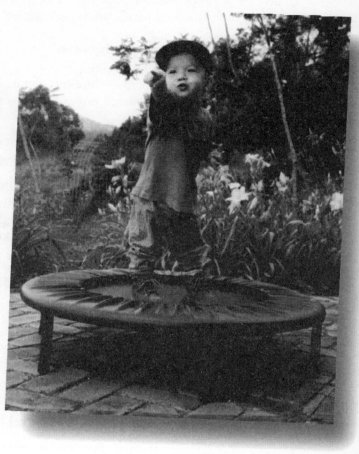

"Please don't buy us kids cheapo trampolines. Only quality materials and good service will give us years of healthy use. Bouncing gently on the trampoline is the best exercise for all ages. Keep your lymph pumping and your eyes moving."—Aerro

Two year warranty on the Vitalizer itself… lifetime guarantee on the Australian steel frame.

Help your child to perfect eyesight — EyeSongs on audio cassette

We all love to singalong with old tunes and new. 32 vision improvement songs and 22 games on audio cassette. Keep Nose Pencils movin' and all hearts groovin'.

Order these indispensable 'visual aids' today with coupon on the next page or contact: Janet Goodrich Centre, 12 Crystal Waters Village MS16, Maleny, Queensland 4552 Australia.

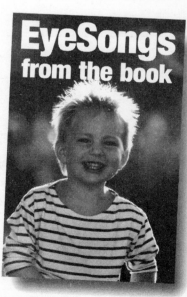

EyeSongs from the book

Become a Janet Goodrich Method Vision Teacher...

Help children and grown-ups recover their eyesight without glasses. You'll have a satisfying career either full or part-time seeing dull eyes light up again with life energy and clarity. If you are dreaming of a job where you relax as well as your students, kindly tick the appropriate box below. We will send you the Certified Instructor information and application package.

THE JANET GOODRICH
Method ‹Natural Vision Improvement›

Easy order form (copy or cut out this page)

Yes. I wish to order the following for my family:

(All prices except for trampoline include shipping and handling within Australia only as of 1996. For other countries and/or updated prices please send a fax or enquiry letter to the address below.)

- ❏ The **VITALIZER** mini-trampoline **$280.00** (Freight to capital cities: $21. Country: $44. N.T. and Tas: $58.)
- ❏ **EyeSongs audio cassette**. Adults will singalong too! **$22.95** Quantity ❏
- ❏ The **6-pack Audio Cassette Album.** 11 vision games and colour visualisations with beautiful music, 3 hours for adults and older children. Includes eyecharts. **$79.95**
- ❏ The full-colour **Eagle Eye Poster** (laminated). Designed by Janet with six vision games at the bottom. Includes explanatory booklet. Great for kids at desks and computers. Size 83 x 56cm. **$43.95**

Please send the following FREE information

- ❏ Pin-holes for children and adults
- ❏ Lectures and seminars with Janet Goodrich for children and adults
- ❏ List of Certified Goodrich Method Teachers
- ❏ Instructor Training Courses (Australia and Germany)
- ❏ Natural Vision Improvement Product Catalogue

Please Print Clearly   Total Amount **$**

Method of Payment: ❏ Cheque ❏ Money Order ❏ Visa ❏ Mastercard ❏ Bankcard

Name: _____

Address: _____

_____

City: _____ State: _____ Post Code: _____

Phone: Day (   )_____ Eve (   )_____ Fax: (   )_____

Card #: __ __ __ __ - __ __ __ __ - __ __ __ __ - __ __ __ __   Exp ___ / ___

Signature: _____
Credit card orders must be accompanied by a signature.

Important: Payment must be made in Australian currency.

✉ Post order to: ☎ 24 hr Fax for fastest service:

Janet Goodrich Centre   **Australia Fax:**
12 Crystal Waters   **OR**   **(074) 94-4673***
MS 16 Maleny, 4552 QLD   **International Fax:**
Australia   **61 74 94-4673***

Thank you for your order!
enquiries please phone (074) 94-4657, 9-12am, 2-5pm Est.

*After October 1996, Phone: (07) 5494-4657 Fax (07) 5494-4673 [61 7 5494-4673].